D1124576

# MRI of the Brain

# MRI of the Brain
## Normal Anatomy and Normal Variants

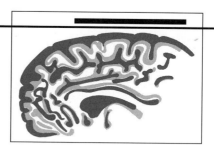

**Vimal H. Patel,** MB, BS, DMRD, FAIS, DNBR, MD
Diplomate, *National Medical and Radiology Board*
Clinical Radiology and Research Scholar
*Neuro and Cross-sectional Imaging*
*McMaster University and Medical Center*
*Hamilton, Ontario, Canada*

**Lawrence Friedman,** MBBch, FFRAD (D) SA, FRCPC, FACR
Director, *Diagnostic Imaging, Guelph General Hospital*
Clinical Professor, *Guelph University, Guelph, Ontario*
Clinical Associate Professor, *McMaster University*
Previous Director, *Neuro and Skeletal Imaging*
*McMaster University and Medical Center*
*Hamilton, Ontario, Canada*

## W. B. Saunders Company
*A Division of Harcourt Brace & Company*
Philadelphia   London   Toronto   Montreal   Sydney   Tokyo

**W. B. SAUNDERS COMPANY**

*A Division of Harcourt Brace & Company*

The Curtis Center
Independence Square West
Philadelphia, Pennsylvania 19106

**Library of Congress Cataloging-in-Publication Data**

Patel, Vimal H.
    MRI of the brain : normal anatomy and normal variants / Vimal H.
Patel, Lawrence Friedman.
        p.   cm.
    ISBN 0-7216-6945-X
    1. Brain—Magnetic resonance imaging.   I. Friedman, Lawrence, MD.
II.  Title.
    [DNLM: 1.  Brain—anatomy & histology.   2.  Magnetic Resonance
Imaging.   WL 141 P295m 1997]
    QM455.P376   1997
    611'.81—dc20
    DNLM/DLC
                                                                96-41701

MRI OF THE BRAIN:
NORMAL ANATOMY AND NORMAL VARIANTS                    ISBN 0-7216-6945-X

Copyright © 1997 by W. B. Saunders Company

All rights reserved. No part of this publication may be reproduced or transmitted in any form or by any means, electronic or mechanical, including photocopy, recording, or any information storage and retrieval system, without permission in writing from the publisher.

Printed in the United States of America

Last digit is the print number:     9    8    7    6    5    4    3    2    1

Qm
455
P376
1997

To my adorable and encouraging parents Harihar and Devyani,
brothers Raj and Bipin, sisters Hemu, Vidhya, and (late) Meena

**V. H. P.**


To my wife Elaine for her enduring love and support,
To my children Talia, Romy, and Saul, who gave meaning to love, and
To my parents for their unconditional love

To Vimal H. Patel, a most productive, outstanding, and endlessly
hardworking, distinguished radiologist and scientist, whose energy,
enthusiasm, and pursuit of excellence were the major factors in the
production of this atlas

To all the residents and fellows I have taught and who in turn
taught me

From darkness to light
Like the relay runner
I merely pass on

The torch of enduring knowledge
Given to me
By so many great teachers

In the hope that one day
The student shall return
To teach the teacher

In the evolution
Of eternal knowledge for all

So that

The patient may ultimately benefit

**L. F.**

# Foreword

It is a pleasure to congratulate Vimal Patel on completion of this atlas of MRI of the normal adult brain. The work provides a detailed and easy to follow reference that will be of value to all who must interpret MR imaging scans. It should prove useful to residents learning their neuroanatomy and to more experienced radiologists who require a reference work, for whom the section on normal anatomic variations is particularly intended.

Vimal Patel came to Canada after ten years of practicing radiology in Bombay with superb ultrasound skills. He rapidly acquired a love for neurological imaging and the study of anatomy and anatomic variations. His dedication to radiology has been an inspiration, and his commitment to the specialty is total. It has been a pleasure and a privilege to have him with us for the past four years at McMaster University. He has shown the same energy, care, and attention to detail in his departmental work that he has put into the illustrations in this book.

This book represents countless evenings and weekends spent collecting material and analyzing images, and our residents, fellows, and faculty will benefit for years to come.

**Giles W. Stevenson, MBch, FRCR, FRCPC**
Professor and Chair, Department of Radiology
McMaster University
Hamilton, Ontario, Canada

# Foreword

Theodore Keats summarized the situation very well when he said that "the problem of normal variation is a lifelong one for the radiologist." With each new modality, radiologists have had to contend with normal variants due to technical factors, anatomy, or drugs used. An ongoing need exists for delineation of normal anatomy and its variants; as the technology improves, the need obviously remains to show previously described information or document normal anatomy with better quality images. As has been found in all radiologic imaging, better understanding of the variants is gained from experience. This textbook was inspired by two critically acclaimed exhibits at RSNA. It draws on years of cumulative experiences, not only of the radiologists writing it, but also of the many radiologists who have, over the years, described both normal anatomy and variants. It illustrates and summarizes current knowledge of normal anatomy of the brain and its borderlands, utilizing high-detail images with concise text in point format as needed, to guide even the most inexperienced student through the vagaries of normal magnetic resonance (MR) imaging anatomy. Despite rapidly changing technology in MR, any book such as this, dealing with normal anatomy and variants, will always be useful. With the high-quality images in the book, it is hoped that this work will remain valid for years, even when MR imaging has plateaued.

**Donald H. Lee, MB, Bch, FRCPC**
Associate Professor, Department of Diagnostic Radiology and
Clinical Neurological Sciences
The University of Western Ontario
London, Ontario, Canada

# Preface

In this book we look at the complex anatomy of the brain viewed through magnetic resonance (MR) imaging using a systematic step-by-step approach. The book is divided into 19 chapters. For each region of the brain, a concise text is arranged in point format, which is easy to understand and remember at any level from first-year medical students to consultant physicians. To make it simpler, we employ flow charts and tables in most chapters. Corresponding anatomic structures have been shown in the sagittal, coronal, and axial thin-section (3 to 5 mm) MR images, acquired on a 1.5-tesla GE MR unit. To enhance the anatomic detail of each structure, the MR inversion recovery (FMPIR) images are printed using inverse video settings. We observe this approach throughout the book. Anatomic structures that are very minute or difficult to appreciate even on high-resolution thin-section MR images are explained in the text. The final chapter on normal variations is based on a collection of cases made over the past six years at our institution.

With this text atlas, we attempt to demonstrate in detail the anatomic information and variations important for the correct interpretation of brain MR images. Although other expensive anatomic atlases exist, it is our belief that there is a need for a publication based on the combination of precise three-dimensional MR images with relevant text in point format and important anatomic variations that must be known in daily practice. The idea was born from the joint success of two projects, both presented at the RSNA annual meetings in 1993 and 1994. Following the success of these educational projects, we obtained an unbelievably positive response from residents, fellows, and staff radiologists. In the progress of these events, we decided to produce a relatively inexpensive combined work useful to medical students, clinical and radiology residents and fellows, neurologists, neurosurgeons, and other physicians.

A work of this type required meticulous preparation of the concise text and the MR images for normal structures and their variants. Unless one has considerable knowledge of the normal structures and variations provided by MR imaging, missed diagnosis or misdiagnosis will result. This text represents ten years of experience teaching neuroanatomy, 36 months of preparation of the exquisite MR images for normal anatomy, and more than six years of painstaking collection of normal variations. Although there were moments of considerable fatigue, we maintained our energy and enthusiasm throughout because of our strong belief that knowledge of anatomy and variations, above all else, is essential for the correct analysis of magnetic resonance images. Indeed, we profited immensely from the information gained during the hours of examining the brain not only with imaging modalities but also with anatomic specimens. It is our hope that the reader, at any level, who studies this book also will profit from the experience and that he or she will understand, more than before, the considerable challenge and spendid opportunity provided by the remarkable techniques utilizing magnetic resonance.

Any comments and suggestions that might improve this work are welcomed. Your participation is of value and will be considered in future editions.

**Vimal H. Patel, MD**
**Lawrence Friedman, MD**

# Acknowledgments

Certainly it is true that behind our accomplishment and success are the influence and thoughtful processes of most people with whom we have worked. I acknowledge with gratitude and affection the heritage of those who helped me in completion of this project and those who trained me in anatomy, radiology, and in particular, neuroradiology.

At W. B. Saunders Company, Vice-President and Editor-in-Chief of Medical Books, Lisette Bralow, and other editorial staff, including Sandra Valkhoff and Joan Balderstone, for their trust and generosity. Without that this project would never have materialized. Melissa Ray and Joan Sinclair, for editing the manuscript and for production processing, and Sally Grande, for all promotional and sales activities.

Loving and caring MR imaging technologists at the McMaster University Medical Center including Hilda Pope, Karen Lightle, Maureen Nichols, Toni Cormier, Sandra Kosakowski, Jay Needles, Jennifer Giglia, and Carol Awde for providing adequate time to obtain the best quality images for this project.

Lawrence Friedman, for his trust, generous support, and guidance in carrying out not only this project but many other projects in neurological and musculoskeletal CT and MRI.

Extremely supportive Chair of the Radiology Division, Giles Stevenson, McMaster University, for providing ample opportunities and academic time, without which completion of this project would not have been possible.

Janet Darby for periodically mailing the entire manuscript to the publisher, Elaine Hewitt for providing computing and printing facilities, and the other secretarial staff for providing their help and services whenever asked.

McMaster University's audio-visual staff, including Rob, John Sr. and Jr., and Patricia, for producing excellent prints for this entire project.

Former and current staff radiologists and technologists from the Sonography, CT, and General Radiology Divisions, fellow colleagues and residents in the McMaster Radiology Division, and related Chedoke group of Hospitals, for rendering their help and assistance in daily work and in crisis.

A team of neuroanatomy professors, Manu Kothari, Lopa Mehta, and K. D. Desai at King Edward Memorial Medical Center, from whom I learned the basics of neuroanatomy.

The best neurophysiology teachers, Tendulkar and Joglekar at King Edward Memorial Medical Center, from whom I clearly understood the physiologic applications of the nervous system.

Dedicated professor, neuroradiologist, and my role model Ravi Ramakantan, Department of Radiology, King Edward Memorial Medical Center, for teaching the basics of neuroradiology.

My best teachers and friends, Suleman Merchant (Sulee) and Om Tawri, Department of Radiology, L. T. Memorial Medical Center, whose encouragement truly helped in building the academic foundation in radiology.

Most helpful dean, Pragna Pai, at the King Edward Memorial Medical Center, whose generous help allowed me to complete in crisis the toughest residency program.

Truly supportive and encouraging Dean S. S. Deshmukh, L. T. Memorial Medical Center, currently the university's Vice-Chancellor, whose direction and vision helped fulfill this dream.

Colleagues, close friends, residents, and medical students at the King Edward Memorial Medical Center, L. T. Memorial Medical Center for advancing my teaching skills in neuroradiology.

**V. H. P.**

# Contents

# CHAPTER 1

# The Brain

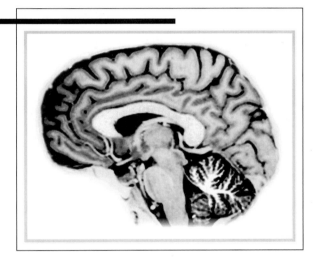

> The brain is the encephalon, the part of the nervous system contained within the cranial vault.

## Major Postembryonic Subdivisions

(Figure **1.1**)

**Prosencephalon:**   Forebrain

**Mesencephalon:**   Midbrain

**Rhombencephalon:**   Hindbrain

## Prosencephalon (Forebrain)

Includes the telencephalon and diencephalon

### Telencephalon

#### *Cerebral Hemispheres*

**Subdivisions:**   Cerebral cortex, or gray matter

White matter:  Cerebral commissures

- Anterior commissure
- Corpus callosum
- Hippocampal commissure

Internal capsule

**Contents:**   Lateral ventricles

**Lobes:**   Frontal, parietal, occipital, temporal, insular, limbic, including the olfactory structures

#### *Basal Ganglia*

**Contents:**   Caudate nucleus

Putamen

Globus pallidus

Amygdaloid complex

Figure **1.1**

The brain (encephalon), major divisions, sagittal view.

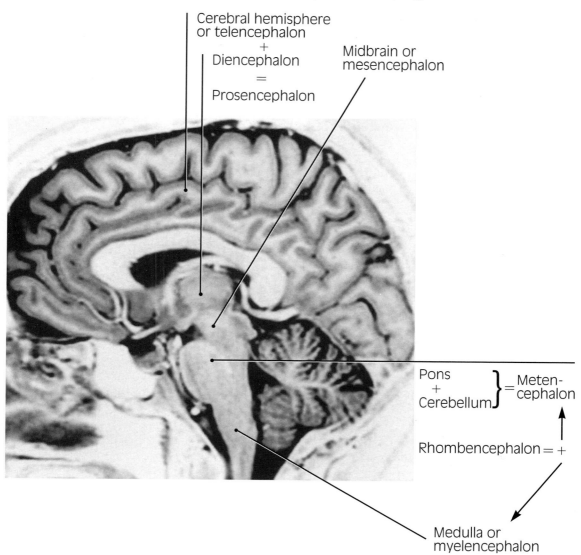

Cerebral hemisphere
or telencephalon
+
Diencephalon
=
Prosencephalon

Midbrain or
mesencephalon

Pons
+
Cerebellum $\Big\}$ = Metencephalon

Rhombencephalon = +

Medulla or
myelencephalon

### Diencephalon

Thalamus

Hypothalamus

Epithalamus

Subthalamus

Third ventricle and related structures

### Mesencephalon (Midbrain)

Parts:  Cerebral peduncles

Interpeduncular fossa with the oculomotor nerve and the posterior perforated substance

Colliculi

Trochlear nerve

Contents:  The aqueduct of Sylvius

### Rhombencephalon (Hindbrain)

Includes the metencephalon and myelencephalon

### Metencephalon

#### *Pons*

Contents:  Trigeminal, abducent, facial, and vestibulocochlear cranial nerves

Structures of the rhomboid fossa

#### *Cerebellum*

Divisions:  Midline vermis

Lateral cerebellar hemispheres

Lobes, lobules, and nodulus

### Myelencephalon (Medulla Oblongata)

Contents:  Pyramid

Olive

Glossopharyngeal, vagus, spinal accessory, and hypoglossal cranial nerves

Tubercles and structures of the rhomboid fossa

# CHAPTER 2

# The Cerebrum

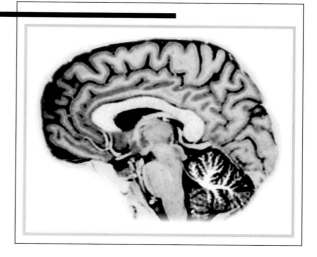

## General Description

(Figure **2.1**)

Contents:   Two cerebral hemispheres

Separation:   Incomplete from each other by the median longitudinal fissure or the interhemispheric fissure and the falx cerebri

Connection:   Connected to each other across the median plane by the corpus callosum

## External Characteristics

Each hemisphere has three surfaces, four borders, three poles, and four major lobes.

### Three Surfaces

Superolateral:   Convex

Related to the cranial vault

Medial:   Flat and vertical

Separated from the corresponding surface of the opposite hemisphere by the falx cerebri and the longitudinal fissure

Inferior:   Irregular

Subdivisions: Anterior—the orbital surface

Posterior—the tentorial surface

A deep cleft, or the stem of the lateral ventricle, separates anterior and posterior surfaces.

Figure **2.1**

The cerebral hemispheres, axial view.

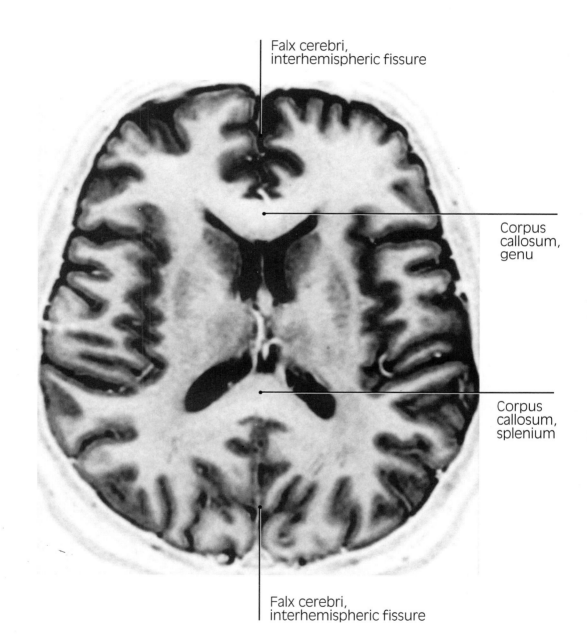

Falx cerebri,
interhemispheric fissure

Corpus
callosum,
genu

Corpus
callosum,
splenium

Falx cerebri,
interhemispheric fissure

## Four Borders

**Superomedial:** Separates the superolateral surface from the medial surface

**Inferolateral:** Separates the superolateral surface from the inferior surface

The anterior part of this border is the superciliary border.

The depression on the inferolateral border, situated about 5 cm in front of the occipital pole, is called the preoccipital notch.

**Medial:** Separates the medial surface from the orbital surface

**Medial occipital:** Separates the medial surface from the tentorial surface

## Three Poles

**Frontal:** Anterior end of the frontal lobe

**Occipital:** Posterior end of the occipital lobe

**Temporal:** Anterior end of the temporal lobe

## Four Major Lobes

(Figure **2.2**)

We better appreciate the lobes on the superolateral surface.

**Frontal:** The largest of all

    Location: Anterior to the central or Rolandic sulcus

        Superior to the lateral or sylvian fissure

**Parietal:** Location: Behind the central sulcus

    Above the lateral fissure

**Temporal:** Location: Ventral to the lateral fissure

**Occipital:** Location: Above the tentorium cerebelli

    Lateral portion: Indistinct boundaries

    Medial portion: Separated from the parietal lobe by the parieto-occipital sulcus

Figure **2.2**

Major lobes, sagittal view.

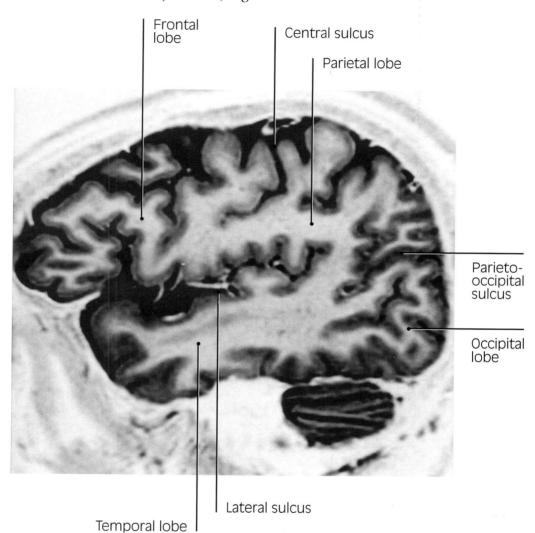

Frontal lobe

Central sulcus

Parietal lobe

Parieto-occipital sulcus

Occipital lobe

Lateral sulcus

Temporal lobe

CHAPTER *3*

# Sulci, Gyri,
# and Fissures

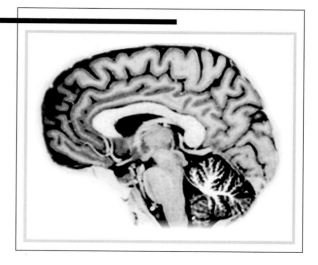

A thin layer of gray matter, the cerebral cortex, covers the surface of each hemisphere. The cortex is folded in a complex fashion so that most of the raised areas or eminences (*gyri*) are separated by depressions or spaces (*sulci*). We apply the term *fissures* to those spaces that are quite deep.

## Main Sulci and Fissures

### Central (Rolandic) Fissure or Deep Sulcus

(Figure **3.1**)

Location:    Roughly perpendicular to the lateral sulcus

Origin:    Slightly behind the midpoint between the frontal and occipital poles at the superomedial border of the hemisphere

Course:    Obliquely downward and forward on the superolateral surface

Ends:    Slightly above the posterior ramus of the lateral sulcus

Function:    To separate the frontal from the parietal lobe

Figure **3.1**

Main sulci, sagittal view.

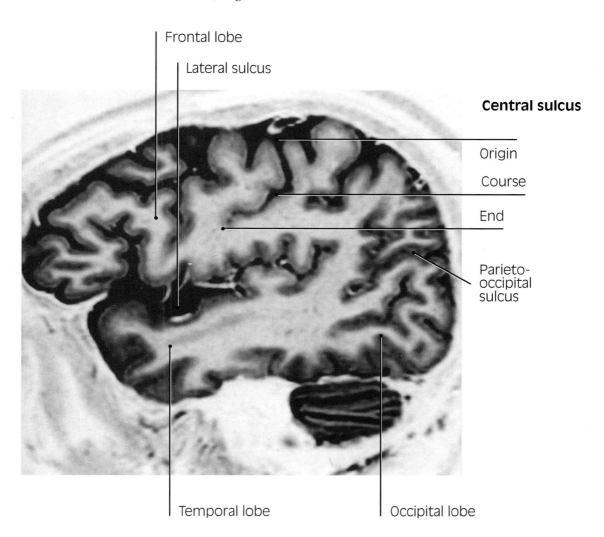

## Lateral (Sylvian) Fissure or Deep Sulcus

(Figures **3.2**, **3.3**, and **3.4**)

Location:   Roughly perpendicular to the central sulcus

Origin:   On the inferior surface

Course:   Posteriorly and upward

Ends:   By dividing into many branches

Branches:   The anterior horizontal and anterior ascending rami extend into the lower part of the frontal lobe.

The posterior ramus, the largest of all, passes backward and upward over the superolateral surface.

Function:   To separate the temporal lobe from the parietal and the frontal lobes

To separate the orbital surface of the frontal lobes from the tentorial part of the inferior surface

> **N O T E**   An important structure deep in the sylvian sulcus is the insula or islet of Reil.

## Parieto-occipital Sulcus

(Figure **3.5**)

Location:   Medial surface. The upper end cuts the superomedial border about 5 cm in front of the occipital pole.

Function:   To separate the parietal lobe from the occipital lobe

# Sulci and Gyri of the Superolateral Surface with Respect to Each Lobe

## Frontal Lobe

(Figure **3.6**)

Precentral sulcus:   Parallel and in front of the central sulcus

Precentral gyrus:   Between the central and precentral sulci

Figure **3.2**

Main sulci, sagittal view.

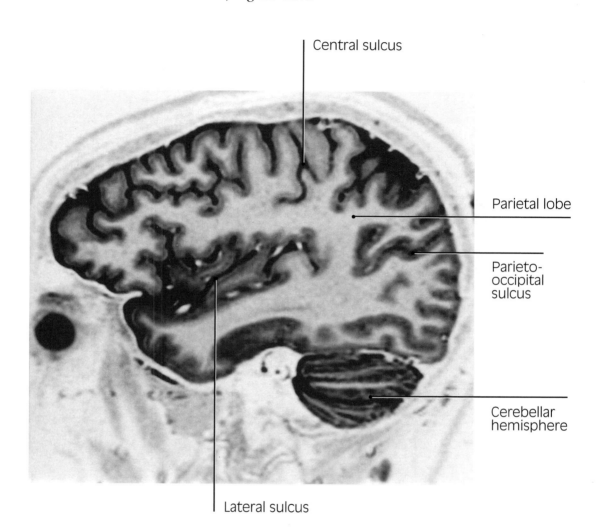

Central sulcus

Parietal lobe

Parieto-occipital sulcus

Cerebellar hemisphere

Lateral sulcus

Figure **3.3**

Lateral sulcus, axial surface.

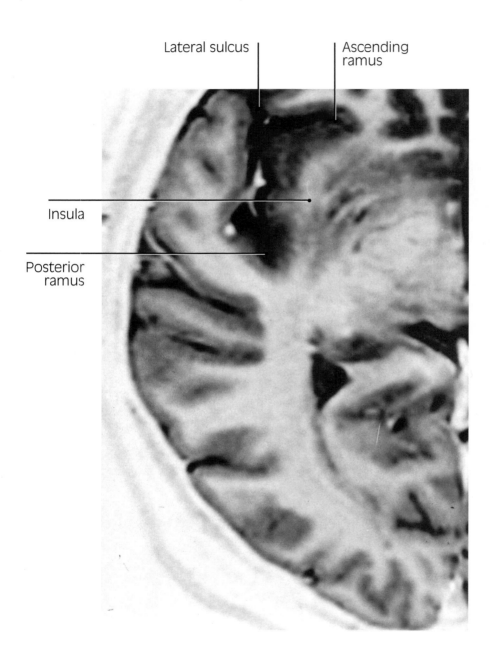

Lateral sulcus

Ascending ramus

Insula

Posterior ramus

Figure **3.4**

Main sulci, coronal view, magnified.

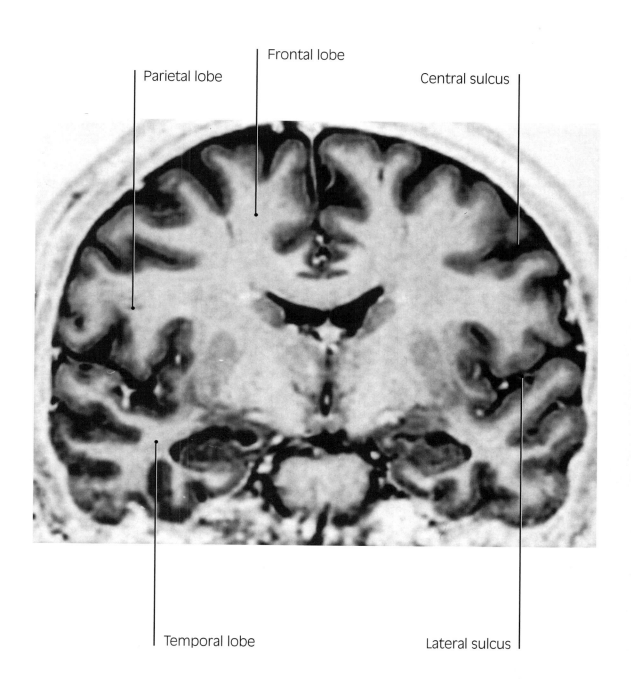

Parietal lobe

Frontal lobe

Central sulcus

Temporal lobe

Lateral sulcus

Figure **3.5**

Main sulci, coronal view, magnified.

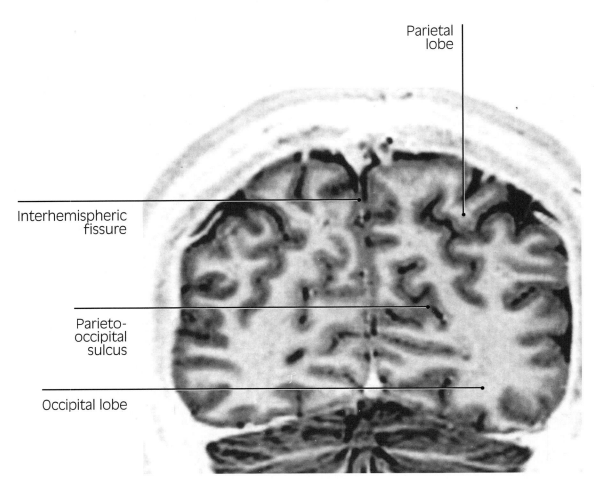

Parietal
lobe

Interhemispheric
fissure

Parieto-
occipital
sulcus

Occipital lobe

Figure **3.6**

Frontal lobe, sulci and gyri, sagittal view.

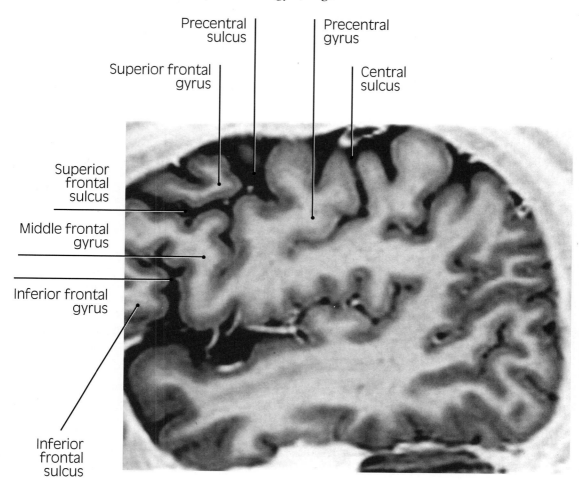

Precentral
sulcus

Precentral
gyrus

Superior frontal
gyrus

Central
sulcus

Superior
frontal
sulcus

Middle frontal
gyrus

Inferior frontal
gyrus

Inferior
frontal
sulcus

### *Primary Motor Area 4 of Brodmann*

- Comprises the precentral gyrus and the anterior wall of the central sulcus.

- One-third of the corticospinal tract occupies area 4 of Brodmann.

- Representation of the body parts is in an orderly fashion from the sylvian fissure to the longitudinal fissure: the jaw, lips, eyelids, thumb, fingers, wrist, elbow, shoulder, hip, knee, ankle, and toes.

- Stimulation of this area results in movements in the opposite half the body.

### *Premotor Area 6 of Brodmann*

- The psychomotor area. Patterns of movement are remembered here.

- Is located just in front of the primary motor cortex and occupies the posterior parts of the superior, middle, and inferior frontal gyri.

- One-third of the corticospinal fibers originate in this area.

### **Area in Front of the Precentral Sulcus**

Divided into the superior, middle, and inferior frontal gyri by the superior, middle, and inferior frontal sulci

(Figures **3.7** to **3.14**)

**Superior frontal gyrus:** Anterior to the precentral sulcus and separated from the middle frontal gyrus by the superior frontal sulcus

**Middle frontal gyrus:** Between the superior and the inferior frontal gyri

**Inferior frontal gyrus:** Anterior to the precentral sulcus and inferior to the middle frontal gyrus

The anterior, horizontal, and anterior ascending rami of the lateral sulcus subdivide the inferior frontal gyrus into the pars orbitalis, pars triangularis, and pars opercularis.

Figure **3.7**

Frontal lobe, sulci and gyri, sagittal view, magnified.

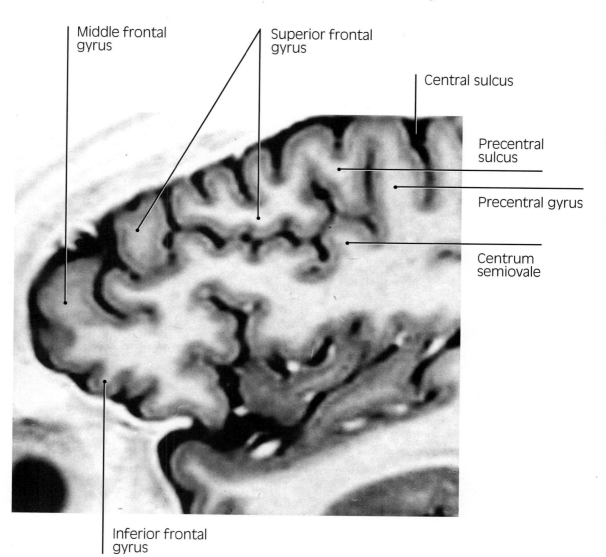

Figure **3.8**

Frontal lobe, sagittal view, magnified.

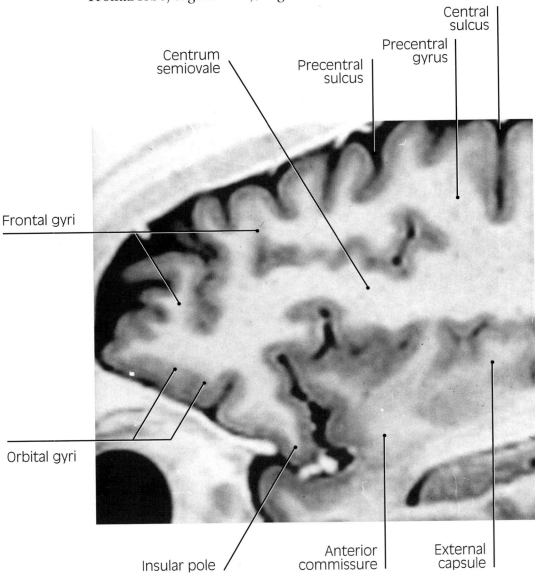

Figure **3.9**

Frontal lobe, sagittal view magnified.

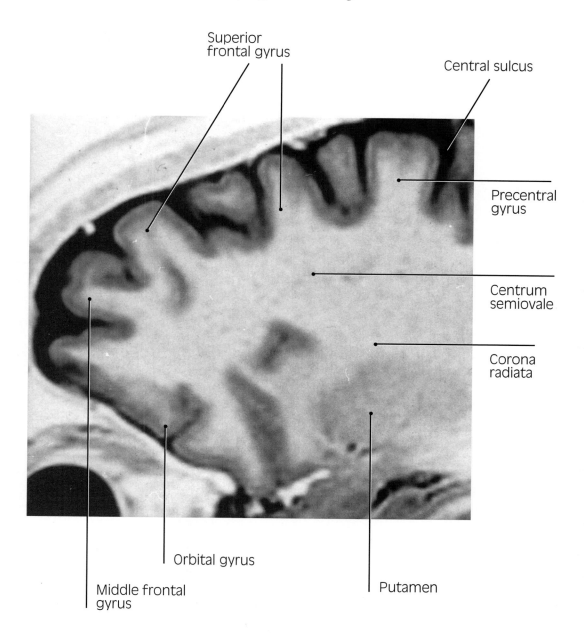

Superior
frontal gyrus

Central sulcus

Precentral
gyrus

Centrum
semiovale

Corona
radiata

Orbital gyrus

Putamen

Middle frontal
gyrus

Figure **3.10**

Frontal and parietal lobes, axial view, magnified.

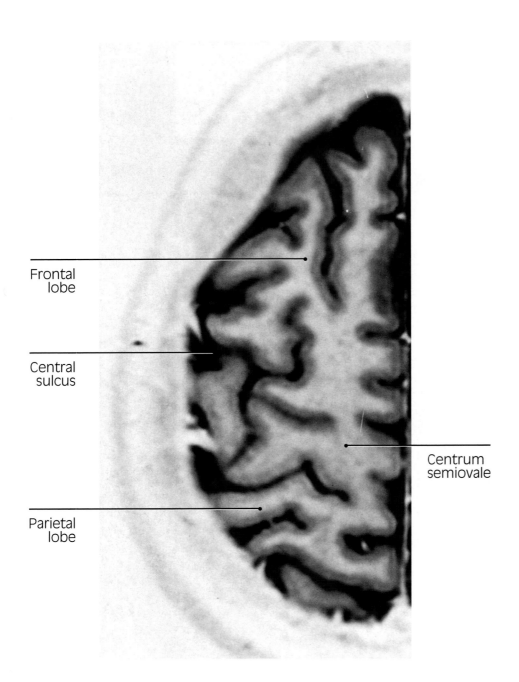

Frontal
lobe

Central
sulcus

Centrum
semiovale

Parietal
lobe

Figure **3.11**

Frontal lobe, axial view, magnified.

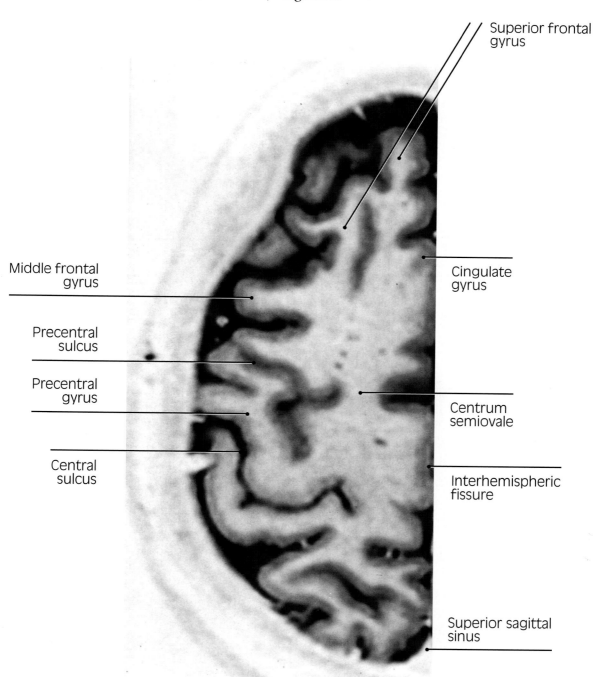

Superior frontal gyrus

Middle frontal gyrus

Precentral sulcus

Precentral gyrus

Central sulcus

Cingulate gyrus

Centrum semiovale

Interhemispheric fissure

Superior sagittal sinus

Figure **3.12**

Frontal lobe, axial view, magnified.

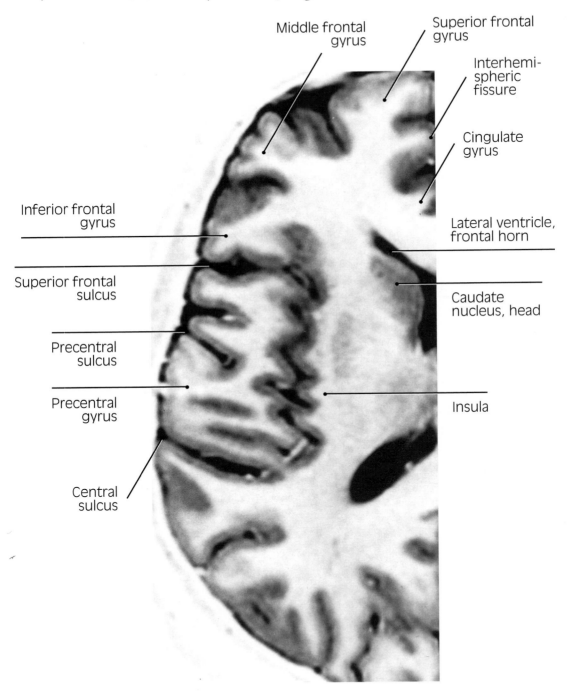

Middle frontal gyrus

Superior frontal gyrus

Interhemispheric fissure

Cingulate gyrus

Inferior frontal gyrus

Superior frontal sulcus

Precentral sulcus

Precentral gyrus

Central sulcus

Lateral ventricle, frontal horn

Caudate nucleus, head

Insula

Figure **3.13**

Frontal lobes, coronal view, magnified.

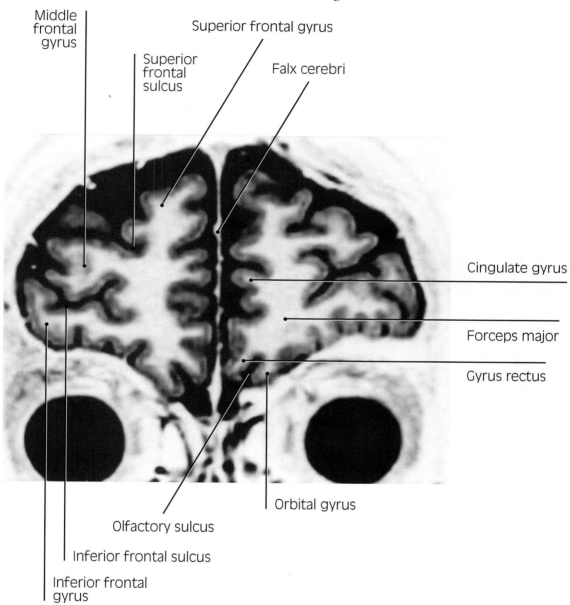

Middle frontal gyrus

Superior frontal sulcus

Superior frontal gyrus

Falx cerebri

Cingulate gyrus

Forceps major

Gyrus rectus

Orbital gyrus

Olfactory sulcus

Inferior frontal sulcus

Inferior frontal gyrus

Figure **3.14**

Frontal lobes, coronal view, magnified.

Middle frontal
gyrus

Superior frontal
gyrus

Cingulate gyrus

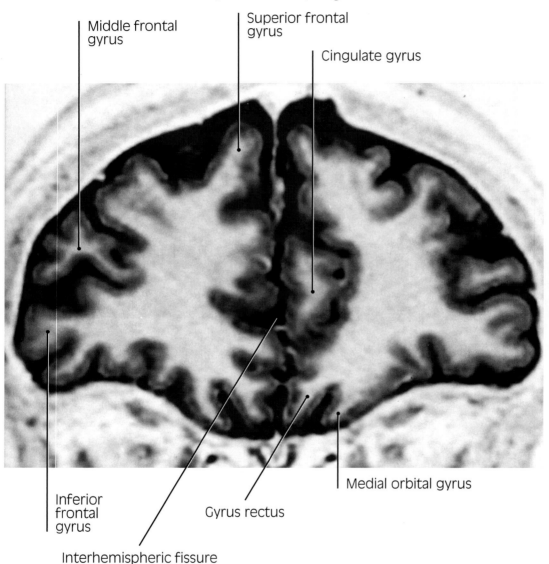

Inferior
frontal
gyrus

Gyrus rectus

Medial orbital gyrus

Interhemispheric fissure

### Area 8 of Brodmann
- Situated in the caudal zone of the middle frontal gyrus
- Stimulation of this area causes conjugate deviation of the eyes toward the opposite side.

### Motor-Speech Area of Broca
- Situated in the inferior frontal gyrus (in the left hemisphere in the right-handed person)
- Lesions of this area cause inability to speak (motor or expressive aphasia).

## Parietal Lobe
(Figure **3.15**)

**Postcentral sulcus:**   Runs parallel and just behind the central sulcus

**Postcentral gyrus:**   Between the central and postcentral sulci

### Primary Somatic Sensory or Somesthetic Area
- Brodmann's Areas 3, 2, and 1.
- The postcentral gyrus and the adjacent posterior wall of the central sulcus.
- Concerned with both superficial and deep sensation.
- Body representation corresponds to the areas of the body in the precentral gyrus.

### Secondary Somatic Sensory or Somesthetic Area
- Located in the parietal lobe posterior to the postcentral gyrus, along the superior border of the sylvian fissure.

### Parietal Lobules

The intraparietal sulcus divides the area behind the postcentral gyrus into the superior and inferior parietal lobules.

(Figures **3.16** to **3.21**)

The inferior parietal lobule is invaded by the upturned ends of the posterior ramus of the lateral sulcus, and of the superior and inferior temporal gyri. They divide the inferior parietal lobule into anterior, middle, and posterior parts.

- Anterior part:

    Supramarginal gyrus just above the temporal lobe

- Middle part:

    Angular gyrus near the apex of the temporal lobe

- Posterior part:

    Merges with parieto-occipital sulcus

**PRACTICAL POINTS**

### Angular Gyrus

- A higher-order association cortex

- Connections with somesthetic visual and auditory association fibers

- Lesions of the angular gyrus may result in severe anomic aphasia, characterized by word-finding difficulties in spontaneous speech.

Figure **3.15**

Parietal lobe, sulci and gyri, sagittal view, magnified.

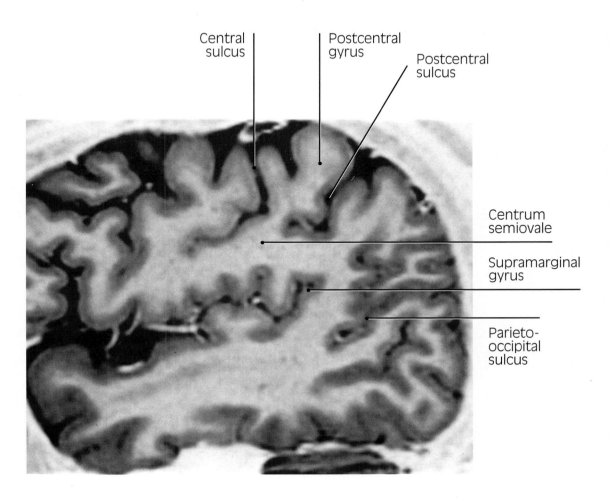

Central sulcus

Postcentral gyrus

Postcentral sulcus

Centrum semiovale

Supramarginal gyrus

Parieto-occipital sulcus

Figure **3.16**

Parietal lobe, sagittal view, magnified.

Postcentral
gyrus

Inferior parietal
lobule

Central sulcus

Parieto-
occipital
sulcus

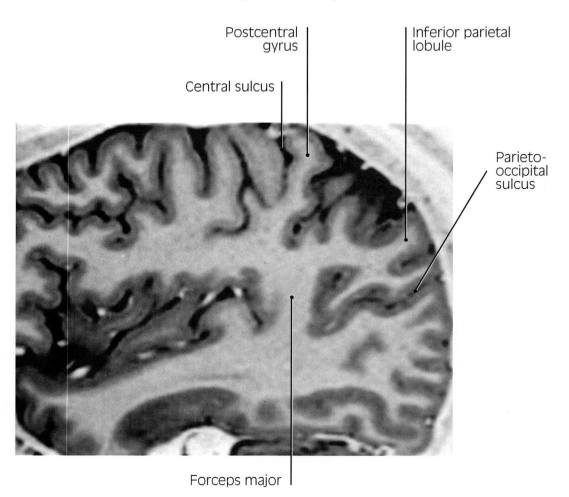

Forceps major

Figure **3.17**

Parietal and occipital lobes, sagittal view, magnified.

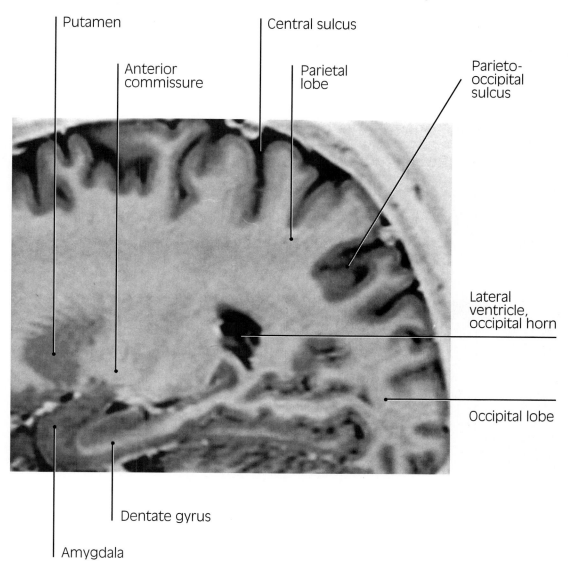

Putamen

Anterior
commissure

Central sulcus

Parietal
lobe

Parieto-
occipital
sulcus

Lateral
ventricle,
occipital horn

Occipital lobe

Dentate gyrus

Amygdala

Figure **3.18**

Parietal lobe, sagittal view, magnified.

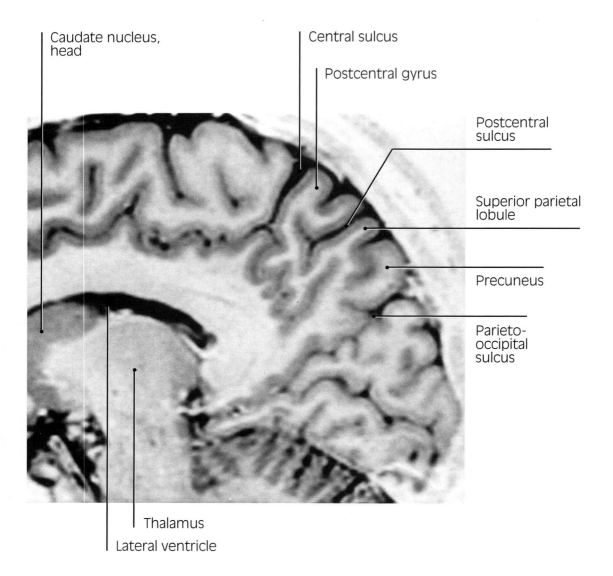

Caudate nucleus, head

Central sulcus

Postcentral gyrus

Postcentral sulcus

Superior parietal lobule

Precuneus

Parieto-occipital sulcus

Thalamus

Lateral ventricle

Figure **3.19**

Parietal lobe, axial view, magnified.

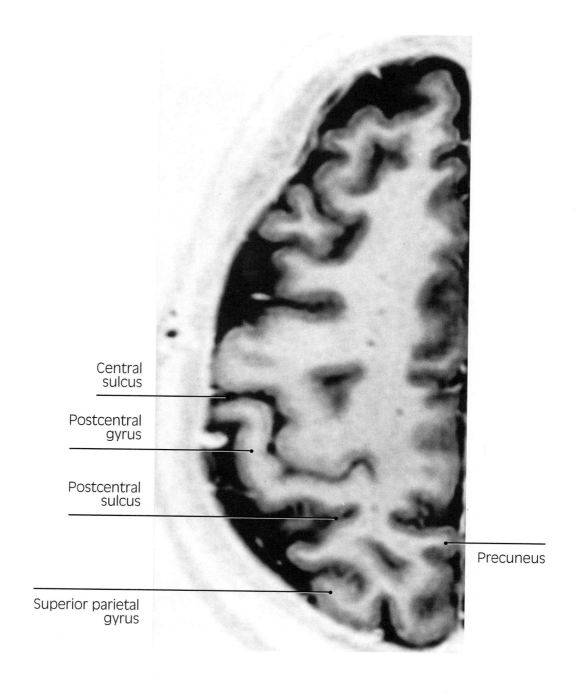

Central
sulcus

Postcentral
gyrus

Postcentral
sulcus

Precuneus

Superior parietal
gyrus

Figure **3.20**

Parietal lobe, axial view, magnified.

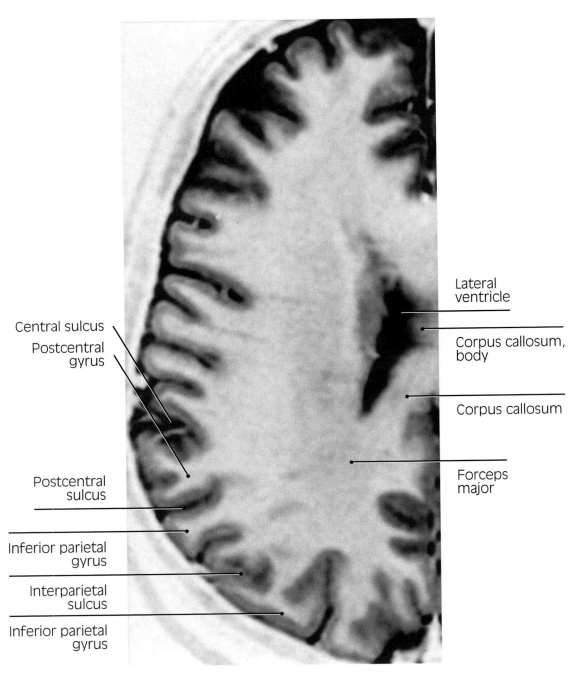

Central sulcus

Postcentral gyrus

Postcentral sulcus

Inferior parietal gyrus

Interparietal sulcus

Inferior parietal gyrus

Lateral ventricle

Corpus callosum, body

Corpus callosum

Forceps major

Figure **3.21**

Parietal lobe, axial view, magnified.

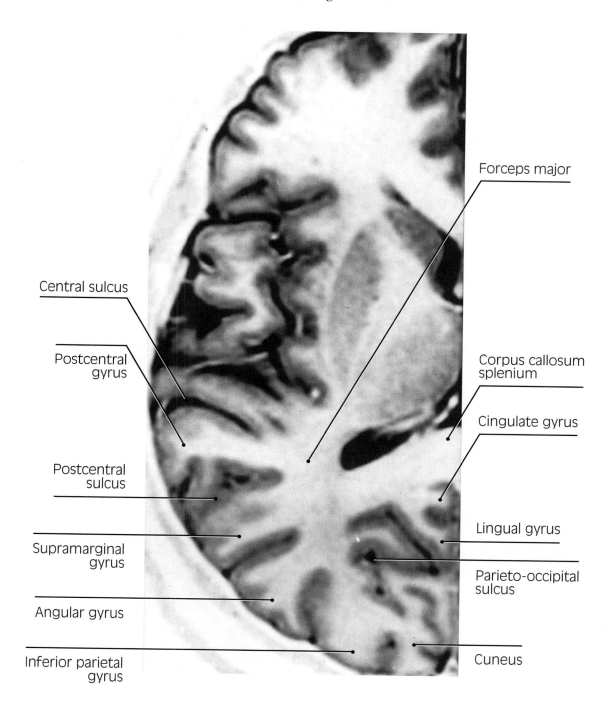

Forceps major

Central sulcus

Postcentral
gyrus

Corpus callosum
splenium

Cingulate gyrus

Postcentral
sulcus

Supramarginal
gyrus

Lingual gyrus

Angular gyrus

Parieto-occipital
sulcus

Inferior parietal
gyrus

Cuneus

## Temporal Lobe
(Figures **3.22** to **3.33**)

The superior and inferior temporal sulci divide the superficial surface of the temporal lobe into the following gyri:

Superior temporal gyrus

Middle temporal gyrus

Inferior temporal gyrus

### Superior Temporal Gyrus

- Anterior superior:

    Comprises the primary, auditory area 41 and some of area 42 of Brodmann.

    Heschl's gyrus lies along the inferior wall of the lateral fissure.

    The secondary, auditory Area 22 and some of area 42 of Brodmann are beside the primary, auditory area in the anterior part of the superior temporal gyrus.

- Posterior superior:

    The auditory association cortex or Wernicke's area

- Lesions of the superior temporal gyrus:

    Cause receptive or sensory aphasia.

### Inferior Temporal Gyrus

- Short-term memory area

Figure **3.22**

Temporal lobe, sagittal view, magnified.

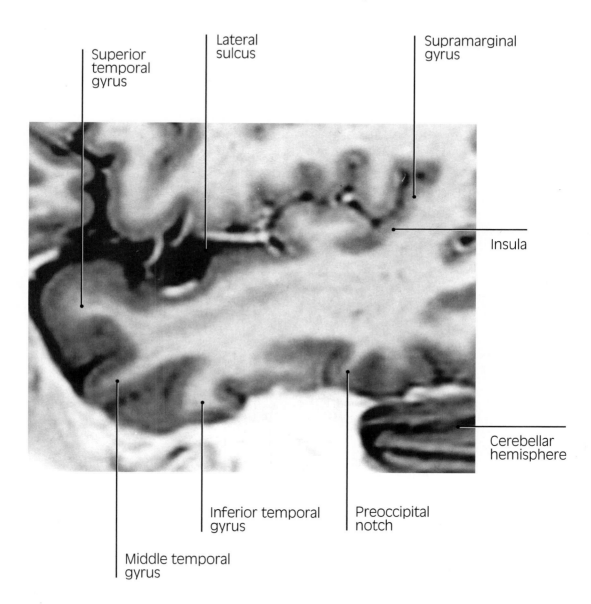

Superior
temporal
gyrus

Lateral
sulcus

Supramarginal
gyrus

Insula

Cerebellar
hemisphere

Inferior temporal
gyrus

Preoccipital
notch

Middle temporal
gyrus

Figure **3.23**

Temporal lobe, sagittal view, magnified.

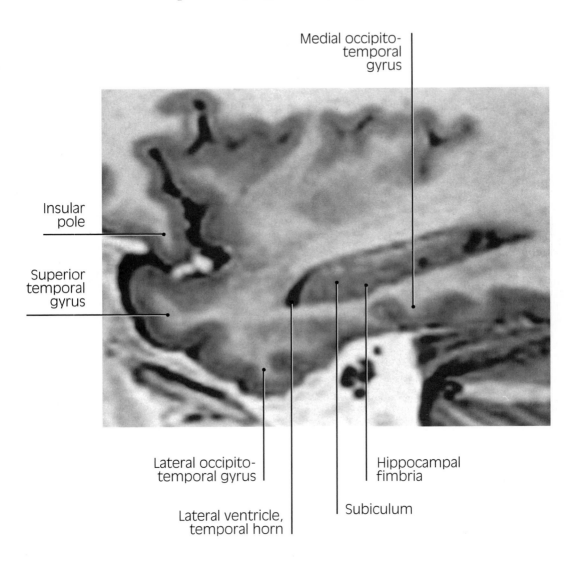

Medial occipito-
temporal
gyrus

Insular
pole

Superior
temporal
gyrus

Lateral occipito-
temporal gyrus

Hippocampal
fimbria

Lateral ventricle,
temporal horn

Subiculum

Figure **3.24**

Temporal lobe, sagittal view, magnified.

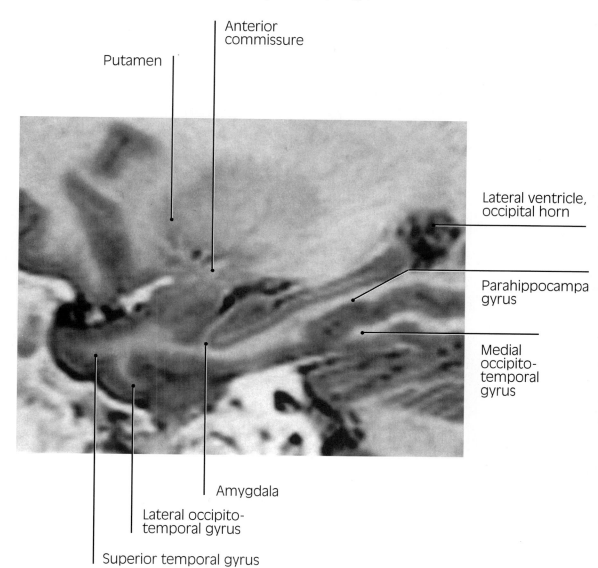

Anterior
commissure

Putamen

Lateral ventricle,
occipital horn

Parahippocampa
gyrus

Medial
occipito-
temporal
gyrus

Amygdala

Lateral occipito-
temporal gyrus

Superior temporal gyrus

Figure **3.25**

Temporal lobe, sagittal view, magnified.

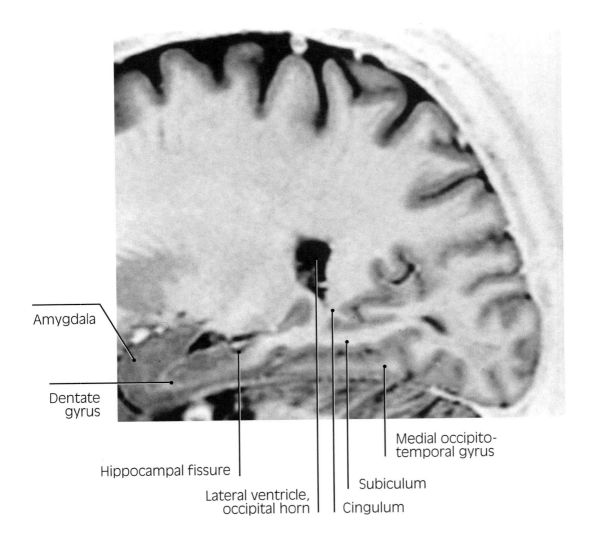

Amygdala

Dentate
gyrus

Hippocampal fissure

Lateral ventricle,
occipital horn

Cingulum

Subiculum

Medial occipito-
temporal gyrus

Figure **3.26**

Temporal lobe, sagittal view, magnified.

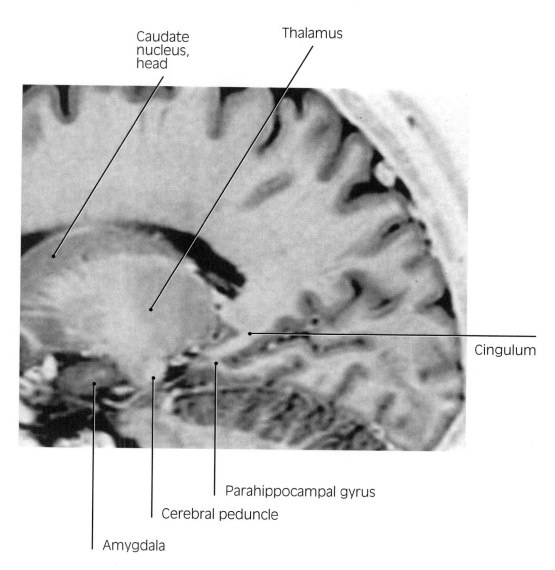

Caudate
nucleus,
head

Thalamus

Cingulum

Parahippocampal gyrus

Cerebral peduncle

Amygdala

Figure **3.27**

Temporal lobe, axial view, magnified.

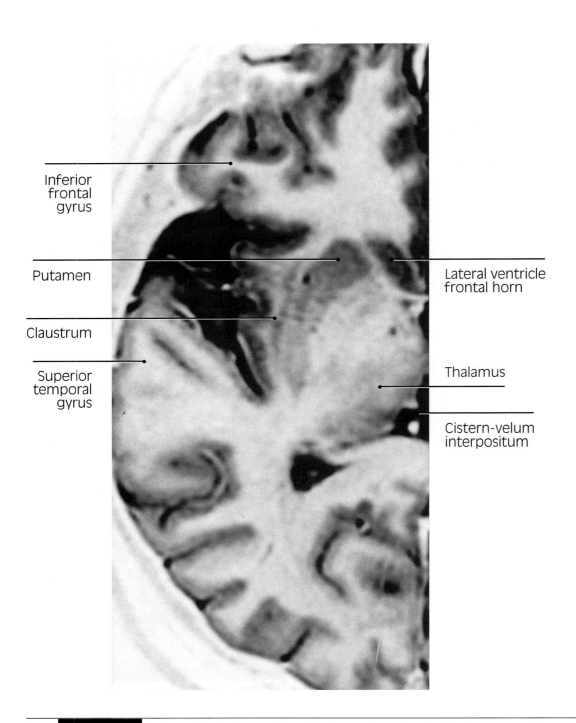

Inferior
frontal
gyrus

Putamen

Claustrum

Superior
temporal
gyrus

Lateral ventricle
frontal horn

Thalamus

Cistern-velum
interpositum

Figure **3.28**

Temporal lobe, axial view, magnified.

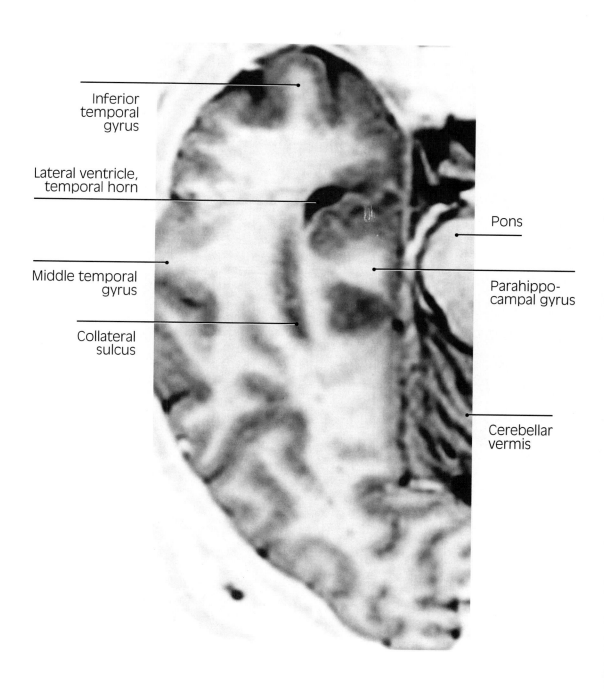

Inferior temporal gyrus

Lateral ventricle, temporal horn

Middle temporal gyrus

Collateral sulcus

Pons

Parahippo-campal gyrus

Cerebellar vermis

Figure **3.29**

Temporal lobes, coronal view, magnified.

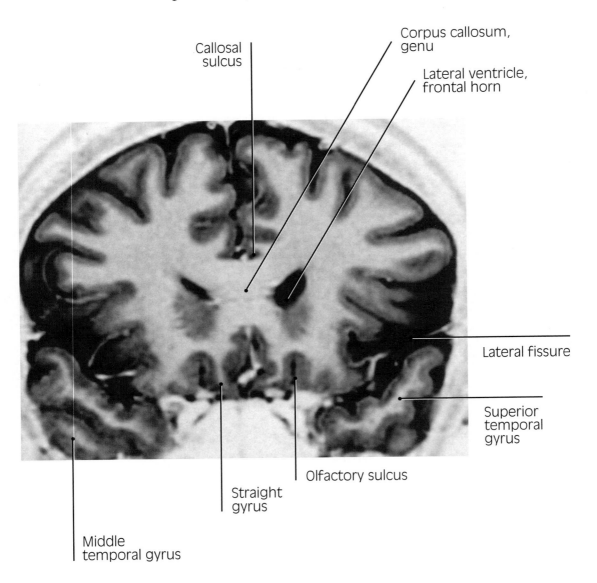

Callosal
sulcus

Corpus callosum,
genu

Lateral ventricle,
frontal horn

Lateral fissure

Superior
temporal
gyrus

Olfactory sulcus

Straight
gyrus

Middle
temporal gyrus

Figure **3.30**

Temporal lobes, coronal view, magnified.

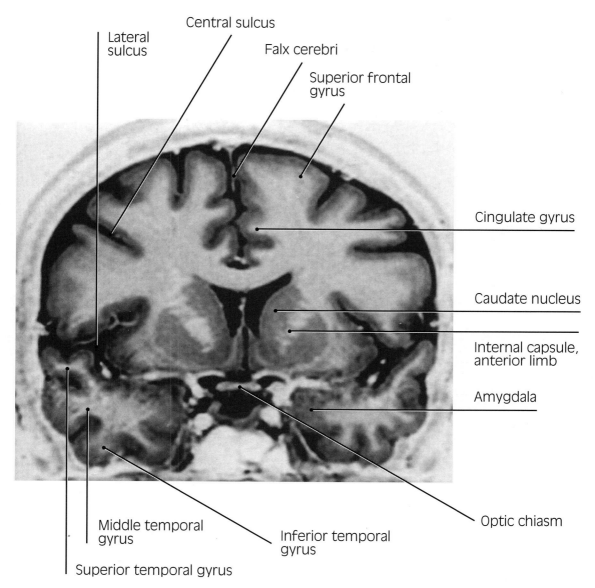

Central sulcus

Lateral sulcus

Falx cerebri

Superior frontal gyrus

Cingulate gyrus

Caudate nucleus

Internal capsule, anterior limb

Amygdala

Optic chiasm

Middle temporal gyrus

Inferior temporal gyrus

Superior temporal gyrus

Figure **3.31**

Temporal lobes, coronal view, magnified.

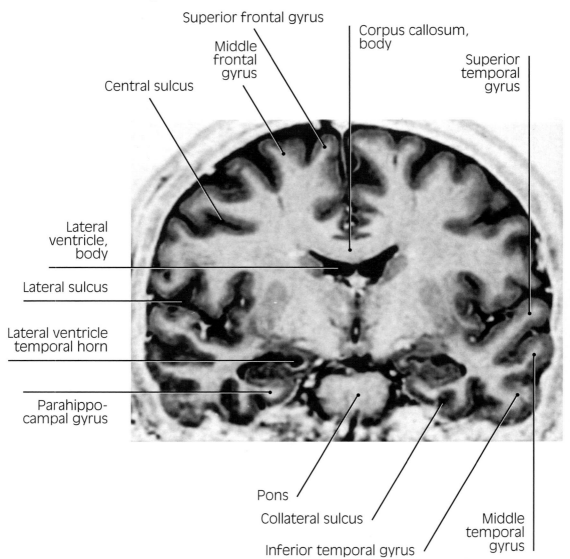

Figure **3.32**

Temporal lobes, coronal view, magnified.

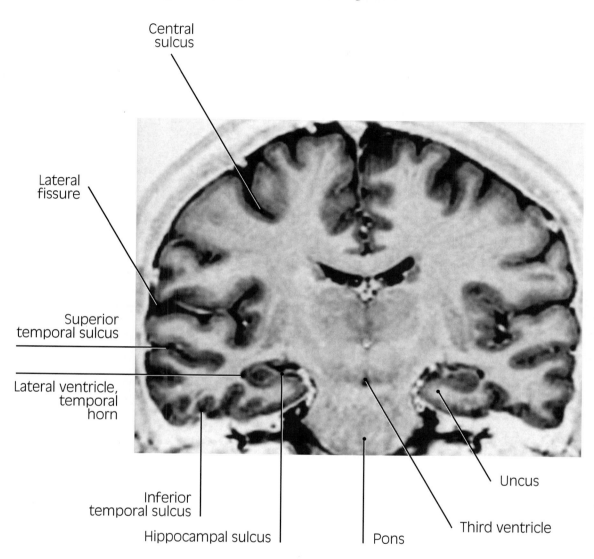

Central
sulcus

Lateral
fissure

Superior
temporal sulcus

Lateral ventricle,
temporal
horn

Inferior
temporal sulcus

Hippocampal sulcus

Pons

Uncus

Third ventricle

Figure **3.33**

Temporal lobes, coronal view, magnified.

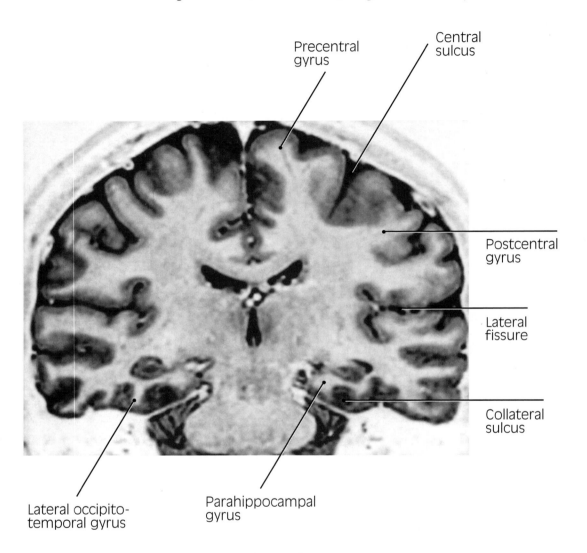

Precentral gyrus

Central sulcus

Postcentral gyrus

Lateral fissure

Collateral sulcus

Lateral occipito-temporal gyrus

Parahippocampal gyrus

## Occipital Lobe
(Figures **3.34** to **3.40**)

Subdivisions by sulci, as follows:

- The lateral occipital sulcus divides this lobe into the superior and inferior occipital gyri.

- The cuneate sulcus separates these gyri from the occipital pole.

- The area around the parieto-occipital sulcus is the arcus parieto-occipitalis. It is separated from the superior occipital gyrus by the transverse occipital sulcus.

## Sulci and Gyri of the Medial Surface
(Figures **3.41** to **3.44**)

### Cingulate Sulcus

Origin:  In front of the genu of the corpus callosum

Course:  Backwards parallel to the upper margin of the corpus callosum

Ends:  A little behind the upper end of the central sulcus

### Cingulate Gyrus

Between the corpus callosum and the cingulate sulcus. The posterior part is bounded above by the suprasplenial sulcus.

### Suprasplenial Sulcus

Above and behind the splenium of the corpus callosum

### Calcarine Sulcus

Origin:  A little below the splenium

Course:  Toward the occipital pole

Branch:  Parieto-occipital sulcus, which reaches the superolateral surface

Figure **3.34**

Occipital lobe, sagittal view, magnified.

Parieto-occipital
sulcus

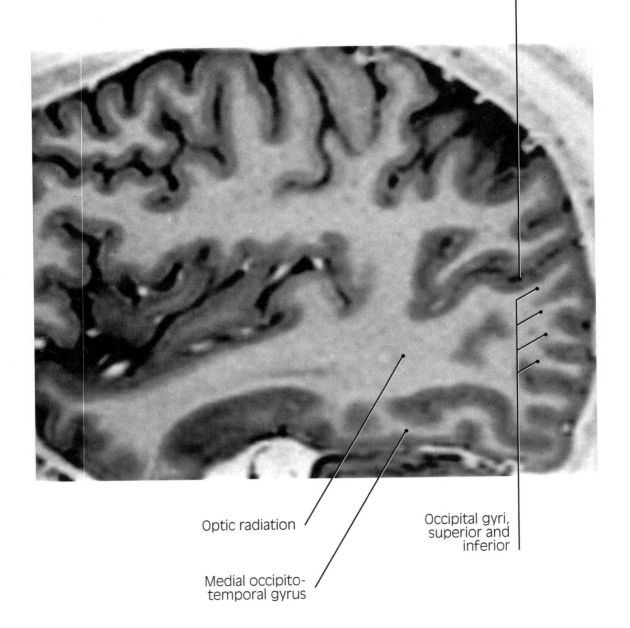

Optic radiation

Occipital gyri,
superior and
inferior

Medial occipito-
temporal gyrus

Figure **3.35**

Occipital lobe, sagittal view, magnified.

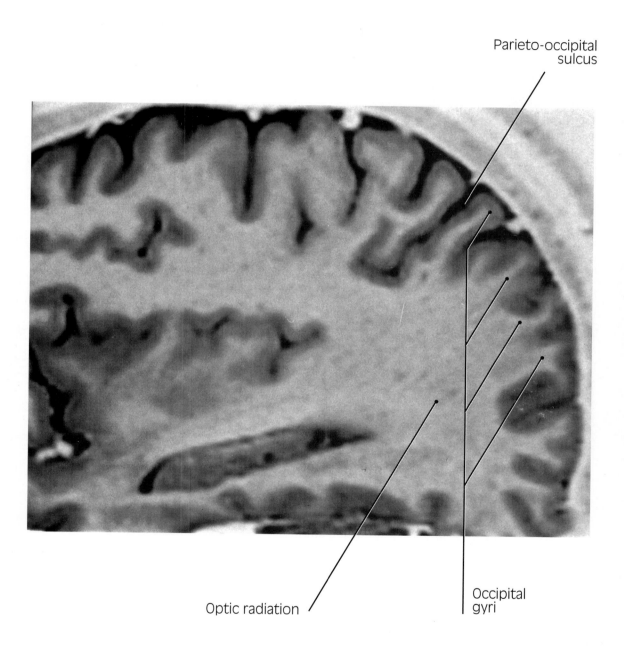

Parieto-occipital
sulcus

Optic radiation

Occipital
gyri

Figure **3.36**

Occipital lobe, sagittal view, magnified.

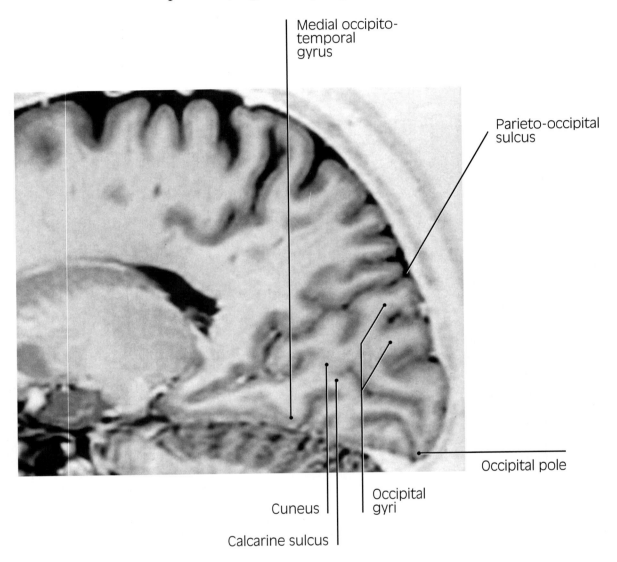

Medial occipito-
temporal
gyrus

Parieto-occipital
sulcus

Occipital pole

Occipital
gyri

Cuneus

Calcarine sulcus

Figure **3.37**

Occipital lobe, axial view, magnified.

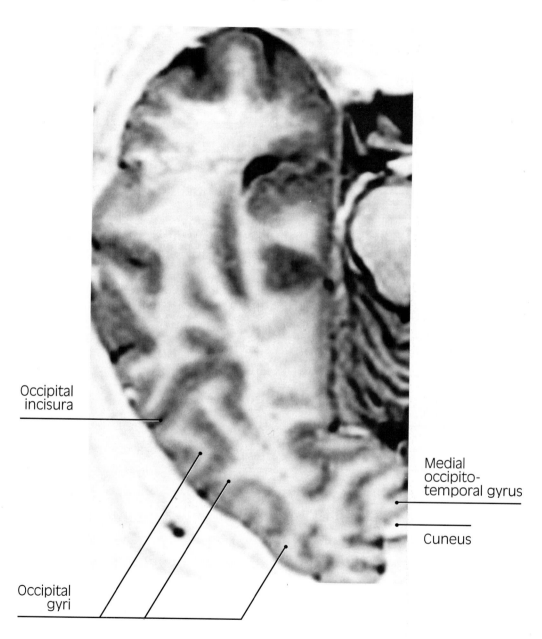

Occipital
incisura

Medial
occipito-
temporal gyrus

Cuneus

Occipital
gyri

Figure **3.38**

Occipital lobe, axial view, magnified.

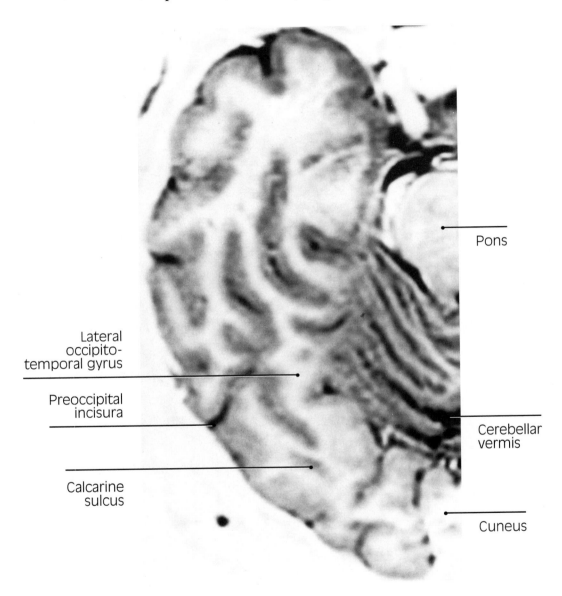

Pons

Lateral
occipito-
temporal gyrus

Preoccipital
incisura

Cerebellar
vermis

Calcarine
sulcus

Cuneus

Figure **3.39**

Occipital lobes, coronal view, magnified.

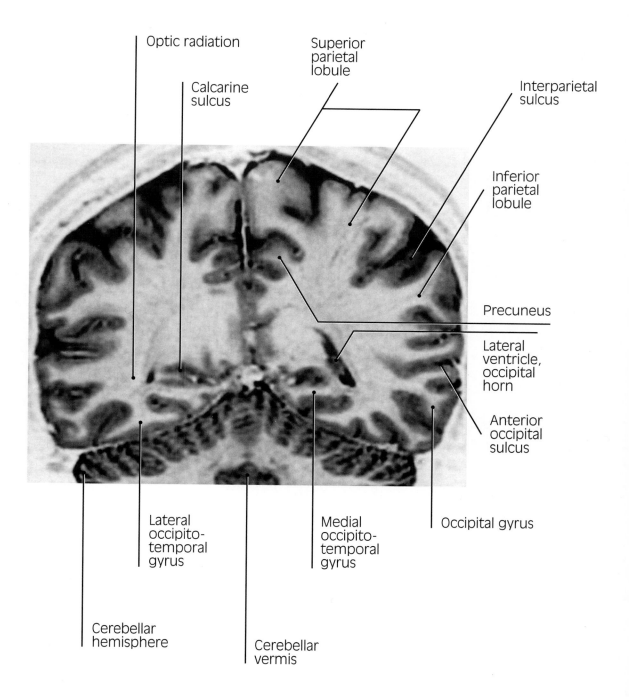

Optic radiation

Calcarine sulcus

Superior parietal lobule

Interparietal sulcus

Inferior parietal lobule

Precuneus

Lateral ventricle, occipital horn

Anterior occipital sulcus

Occipital gyrus

Medial occipito-temporal gyrus

Lateral occipito-temporal gyrus

Cerebellar hemisphere

Cerebellar vermis

Figure **3.40**

Occipital lobe, coronal view, magnified.

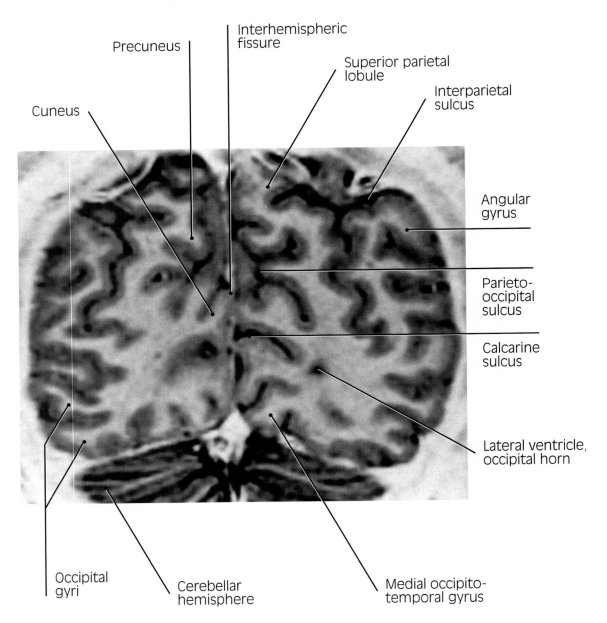

Precuneus

Interhemispheric fissure

Superior parietal lobule

Interparietal sulcus

Cuneus

Angular gyrus

Parieto-occipital sulcus

Calcarine sulcus

Lateral ventricle, occipital horn

Occipital gyri

Cerebellar hemisphere

Medial occipito-temporal gyrus

Figure **3.41**

Sulci and gyri, medial surface, sagittal view, magnified.

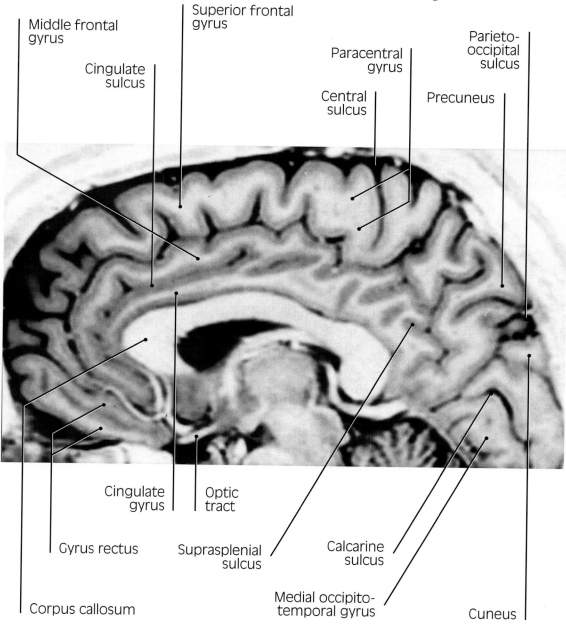

Middle frontal gyrus

Superior frontal gyrus

Parieto-occipital sulcus

Cingulate sulcus

Paracentral gyrus

Central sulcus

Precuneus

Cingulate gyrus

Optic tract

Gyrus rectus

Suprasplenial sulcus

Calcarine sulcus

Corpus callosum

Medial occipito-temporal gyrus

Cuneus

Figure **3.42**

Sulci and gyri, medial surface, sagittal view, magnified.

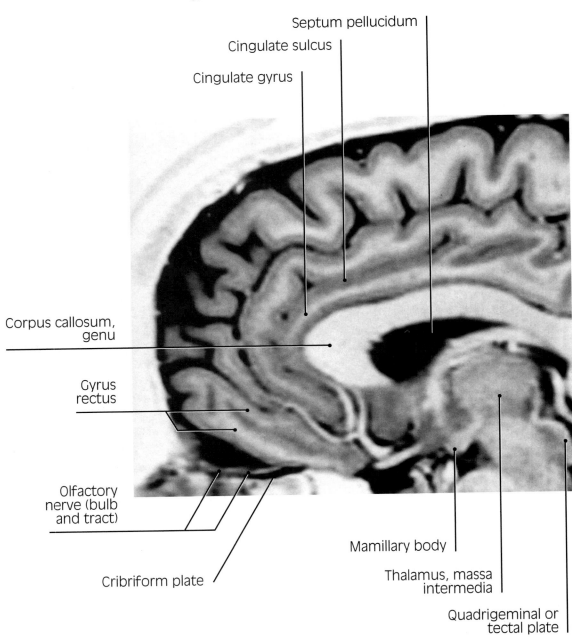

Septum pellucidum

Cingulate sulcus

Cingulate gyrus

Corpus callosum, genu

Gyrus rectus

Olfactory nerve (bulb and tract)

Cribriform plate

Mamillary body

Thalamus, massa intermedia

Quadrigeminal or tectal plate

Figure **3.43**

Sulci and gyri, medial surface, sagittal view, magnified.

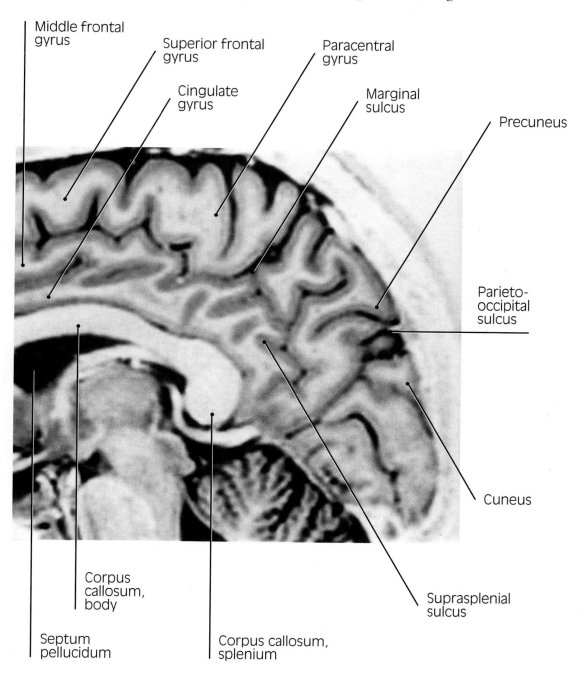

Middle frontal
gyrus

Superior frontal
gyrus

Paracentral
gyrus

Cingulate
gyrus

Marginal
sulcus

Precuneus

Parieto-
occipital
sulcus

Cuneus

Corpus
callosum,
body

Suprasplenial
sulcus

Septum
pellucidum

Corpus callosum,
splenium

Figure **3.44**

Sulci and gyri, medial surface, sagittal view, magnified.

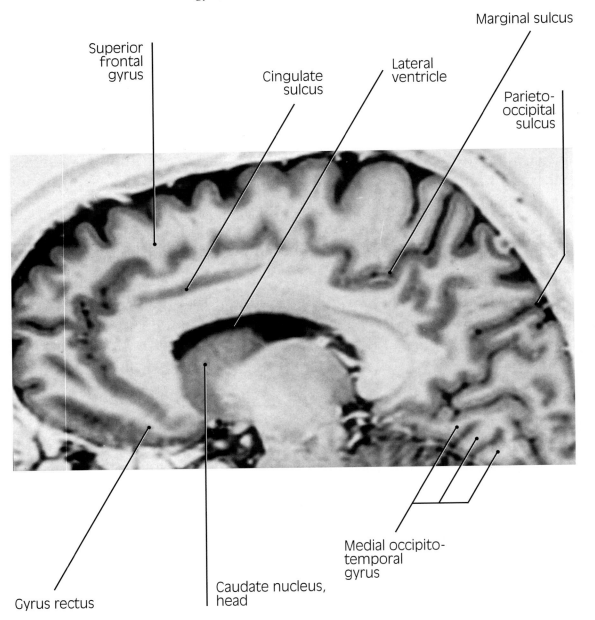

Marginal sulcus

Superior
frontal
gyrus

Cingulate
sulcus

Lateral
ventricle

Parieto-
occipital
sulcus

Gyrus rectus

Caudate nucleus,
head

Medial occipito-
temporal
gyrus

**PRACTICAL POINTS**

- The primary visual area is found along the banks of the calcarine sulcus.

- The secondary visual areas 18 and 19 of Brodmann are near area 17 in the occipital pole.

- The anterior and posterior paraolfactory sulci are a little below the genu of the corpus callosum.

- The paracentral U-shaped gyrus is around the end of the central sulcus.

- The medial frontal gyrus is between the gyrus cingulate and the superomedial border, in front of the paracentral lobule.

- The precuneus is the quadrangular area between the suprasplenial gyrus and the superomedial border.

- The cuneus is the triangular area between the parieto-occipital sulcus above and the calcarine sulcus below.

- The isthmus is a narrow strip between the splenium of the corpus callosum and the stem of the calcarine sulcus.

- The paraterminal gyrus lies just in front of the lamina terminalis.

## Sulci and Gyri on the Orbital Surface

- The olfactory sulcus is parallel to the medial orbital border.

- The gyrus rectus is medial to the olfactory sulcus.

- The H-shaped sulcus divides the orbital surface except the part covering the olfactory sulcus into anterior, posterior, medial, and lateral orbital gyri.

## Sulci and Gyri on the Tentorial Surface

- Two sulci on this surface run anteroposteriorly. The medial sulcus is the collateral sulcus, and the lateral sulcus is the occipitotemporal sulcus. The part medial to the collateral sulcus is the parahippocampal gyrus, and the part lateral to the collateral sulcus is divided into medial and lateral occipitotemporal gyri by the occipitotemporal sulcus.

- The rhinal sulcus is on the medial side of the temporal lobe. The uncus is the part medial to the rhinal sulcus.

CHAPTER *4*

# Diencephalon

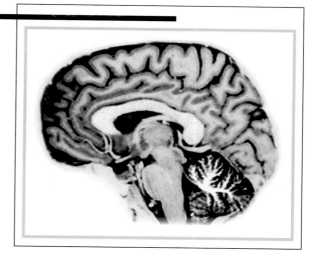

The diencephalon is a midline rostral portion of the brain stem. Its cavity forms the greater part of the third ventricle.

## Relationships

| | |
|---|---|
| **Superior:** | Choroid plexus of the third ventricle |
| | Anterior fornix |
| **Inferior:** | Optic chiasm |
| | Optic tracts |
| | Pituitary stalk |
| | Mamillary bodies |
| **Rostral:** | Foramen of Monro |
| **Caudal:** | Midbrain |
| **Medial:** | Wall of the third ventricle |
| **Lateral:** | Posterior limb of the internal capsule |

## Divisions

The hypothalamic sulcus, extending from the interventricular foramen to the cerebral aqueduct, divides each half of the diencephalon into dorsal and ventral parts. Further subdivisions are as follows:

| | |
|---|---|
| **Dorsal diencephalon:** | Thalamus |
| | Metathalamus |
| | Epithalamus |
| **Ventral diencephalon:** | Subthalamus |
| | Hypothalamus |

## Dorsal Diencephalon

### Thalamus

(Figures **4.1** to **4.3**)

The thalamus is a large mass of gray matter in the lateral wall of the third ventricle and in the floor of the central part of the lateral ventricle. It has anterior and posterior ends and superior, inferior, medial, and lateral surfaces. It bulges posteriorly because of the pulvinar.

Figure **4.1**

Thalamus, sagittal view.

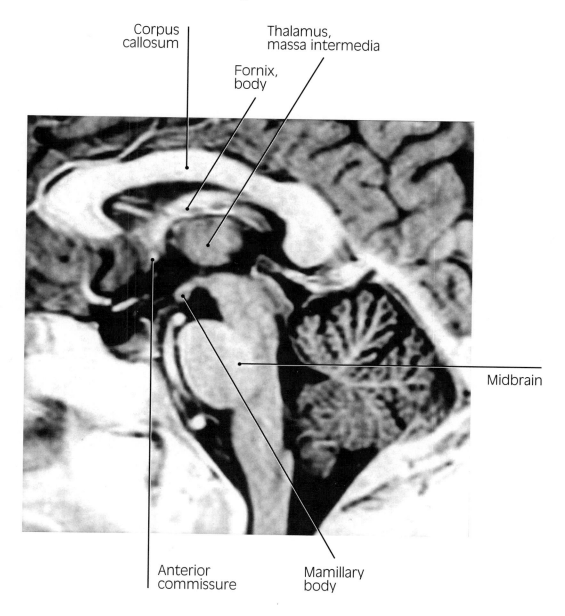

Corpus callosum

Thalamus, massa intermedia

Fornix, body

Midbrain

Anterior commissure

Mamillary body

Figure **4.2**

## Thalamus, sagittal view.

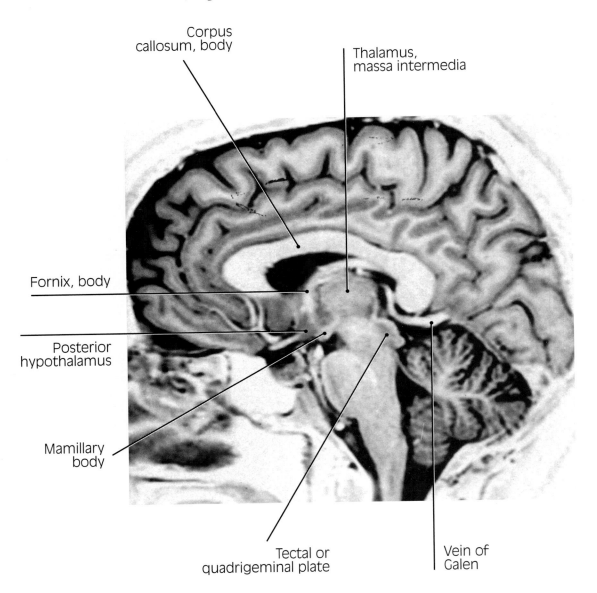

Corpus
callosum, body

Thalamus,
massa intermedia

Fornix, body

Posterior
hypothalamus

Mamillary
body

Tectal or
quadrigeminal plate

Vein of
Galen

Figure **4.3**

Thalamus, sagittal view.

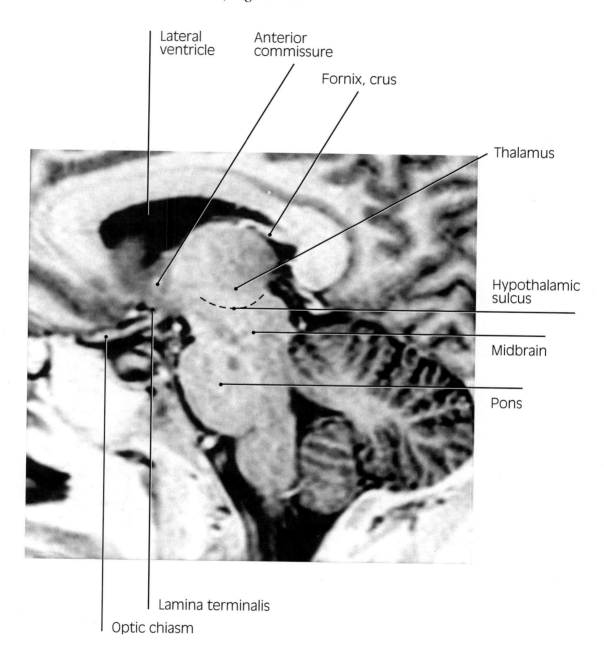

Lateral ventricle

Anterior commissure

Fornix, crus

Thalamus

Hypothalamic sulcus

Midbrain

Pons

Lamina terminalis

Optic chiasm

Anterior end:  Narrow

Forms the posterior boundary of the interventricular foramen

Posterior end:  Expanded, known as the pulvinar

Overhangs the lateral and medial geniculate bodies and the brachium of the superior colliculus

Superior surface:  Lateral ventricular part: Forms the floor of the central part of the lateral ventricle

Medial extraventricular part: Covered by the tela choroidea of the third ventricle

Inferior surface:  Rests on the subthalamus and hypothalamus

Medial surface:  Forms the posterosuperior part of the lateral wall of the third ventricle and connects with the opposite thalamus by the interthalamic adhesion, the massa intermedia

Lateral surface:  Forms the medial boundary of the posterior limb of the internal capsule

## Thalamic Structure and Nuclei

### *Anatomical Divisions*

White matter:  The external medullary lamina covers the lateral surface.

The internal medullary lamina divides the thalamus into three parts: anterior, medial, and lateral.

Gray matter:  Divides and forms several nuclei as follows

(Figures **4.4** to **4.11**)

Figure **4.4**

Thalamus, divisions, sagittal view.

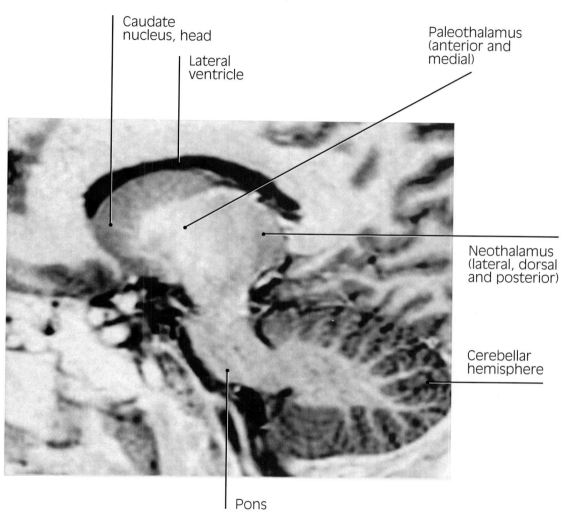

Caudate
nucleus, head

Lateral
ventricle

Paleothalamus
(anterior and
medial)

Neothalamus
(lateral, dorsal
and posterior)

Cerebellar
hemisphere

Pons

| Thalamus | Parts | Nuclei |
|---|---|---|
| Paleothalamus | Anterior group | Part of the Papez circuit |
| | Medial dorsal | Dorsomedial nucleus |
| Neothalamus | Lateral dorsal | Lateral dorsal nucleus |
| | Lateral posterior | Lateral posterior nucleus |
| | Ventromedial | Ventral nuclei: Anterior |
| | | Intermediate |
| | | Posterior: Lateral |
| | | Medial |
| Internal medullary lamina | | Intralaminal nuclei |
| Periventricular gray matter on the medial surface | | Midline nuclei |
| Lateral surface | | Reticular nuclei |

### Functional Divisions
**Cortical relay nuclei:**  Anterior, ventral lateral, and ventral medial
**Sensory relay nuclei:**  Ventral posterior, lateral, and medial
Medial and lateral geniculate bodies
**Association nuclei:**  Lateral and dorsomedial
Midline and intralaminar nuclei

**PRACTICAL POINTS**

**Thalamic lesions:**  Impairment of all sensibilities with maximum involvement of the joint and postural senses

**Thalamic syndrome:**  Disturbances of sensations
Hemiplegia or hemiparesis
Hyperaesthesia
Severe spontaneous pain
Exaggeration of pleasant and unpleasant sensations or feeling

Figure **4.5**

Paleothalamus, nuclei, sagittal view (arbitrary divisions based on available experimental and pathological data and may need to be revised in the future).

(Part of Papez circuit)

Anterior nuclear group

Medial nuclear group

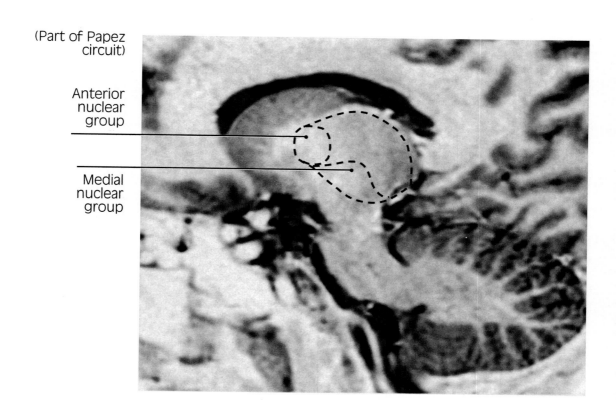

Anterior group: Large anterior medial and dorsal + small anterior ventral

Medial group: Large medial dorsal + a sum of smaller nuclei

Figure **4.6**

Neothalamus, nuclei, sagittal view (arbitrary divisions based on available experimental and pathological data and may need to be revised in the future).

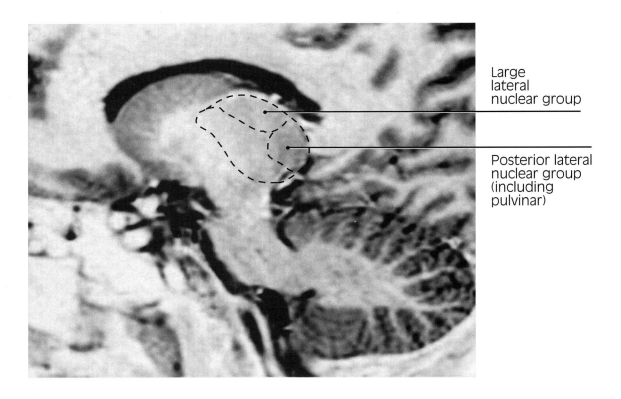

Large
lateral
nuclear group

Posterior lateral
nuclear group
(including
pulvinar)

Lateral group:  Large lateral dorsal and posterior + small
lateral ventral posterior
Posterior group: Large lateral posterior + small lateral ventral posterior
Reticular nuclei on the extreme lateral surface

Figure **4.7**

Thalamus, sagittal view.

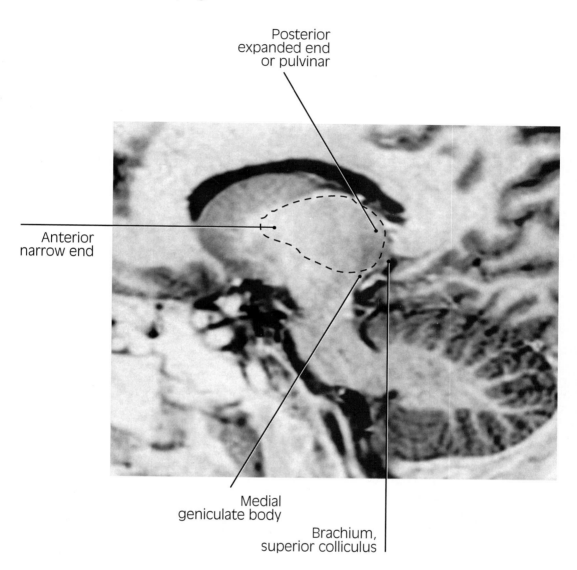

Posterior
expanded end
or pulvinar

Anterior
narrow end

Medial
geniculate body

Brachium,
superior colliculus

Figure **4.8**

Thalamus, axial view, magnified.

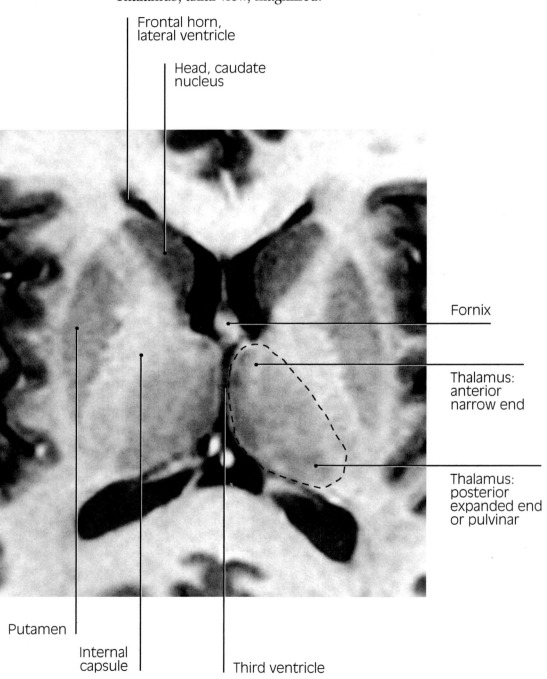

Frontal horn,
lateral ventricle

Head, caudate
nucleus

Fornix

Thalamus:
anterior
narrow end

Thalamus:
posterior
expanded end
or pulvinar

Putamen

Internal
capsule

Third ventricle

Figure **4.9**

Thalamus, divisions, axial view, magnified (arbitrary divisions based on available experimental and pathological data and may need to be revised in the future).

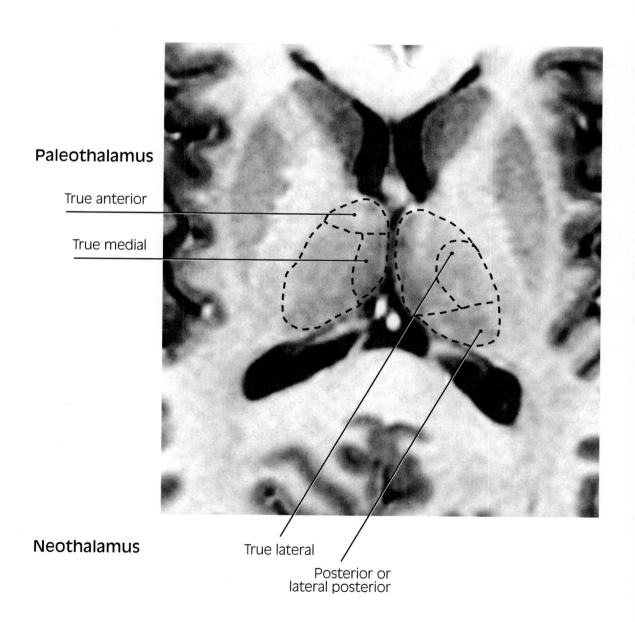

**Paleothalamus**

True anterior

True medial

**Neothalamus**

True lateral

Posterior or
lateral posterior

Figure **4.10**

Thalamus, axial view.

Thalamus                    Thalamus

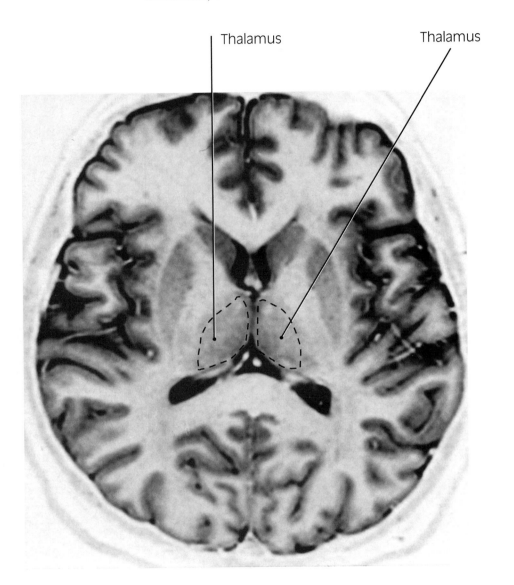

Figure **4.11**

Thalamus, coronal view.

Caudate nucleus | | Thalamus

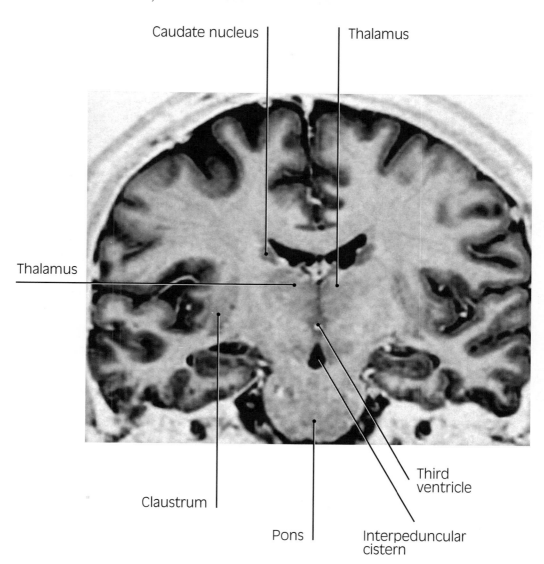

Thalamus

Claustrum |

Pons | 

Interpeduncular cistern

Third ventricle

## Metathalamus

(Figures **4.12** to **4.14**)

Location:   Below the thalamus

Parts:   Medial and lateral geniculate bodies, each side of the midbrain

### Medial Geniculate Body

Shape:   Large, ovoid

Location:   Below the pulvinar of the thalamus

Lateral to the superior colliculus

Connection:   To inferior colliculus via inferior brachium

Function:   Auditory

### Lateral Geniculate Body

Shape:   Small, ovoid

Location:   Below the thalamus

Anterolateral to the medial geniculate body

Partly overlapped by the medial temporal lobe

Connection:   To superior colliculus via superior brachium

Function:   Visual

Figure **4.12**

Metathalamus: sagittal view, magnified.

Caudate
nucleus, head

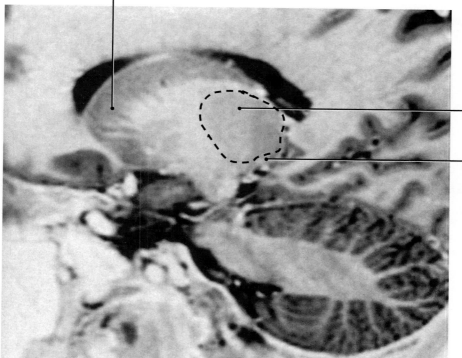

Thalamus

Metathalamus,
medial
geniculate
body

Figure **4.13**

Metathalamus, sagittal view.

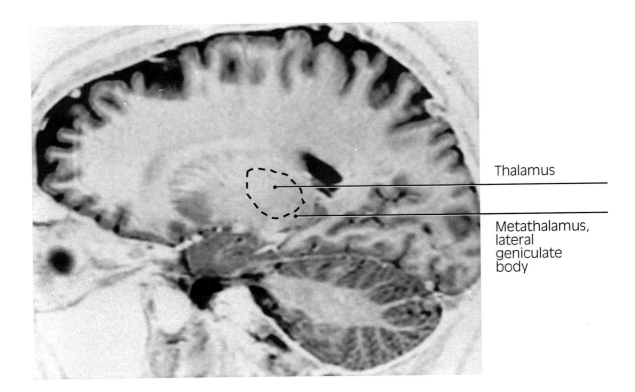

Thalamus

Metathalamus,
lateral
geniculate
body

Figure **4.14**

Metathalamus, coronal view.

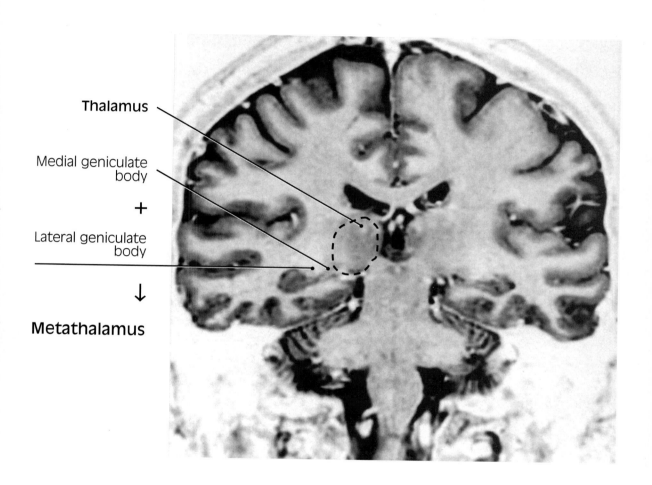

Thalamus

Medial geniculate
body

+

Lateral geniculate
body

↓

**Metathalamus**

## Epithalamus

(Figures **4.15** to **4.18**)

Location:    Caudal part of the roof of the diencephalon

Parts:    Habenular nuclei

Habenular commissure

Posterior commissure

Pineal body

### Habenular Nuclei

Location:    In the floor of the habenular trigone (a small depressed triangular area situated above the superior colliculus and medial to the pulvinar of the thalamus)

Functions:    Part of the limbic system

Figure **4.15**

Epithalamus, axial view.

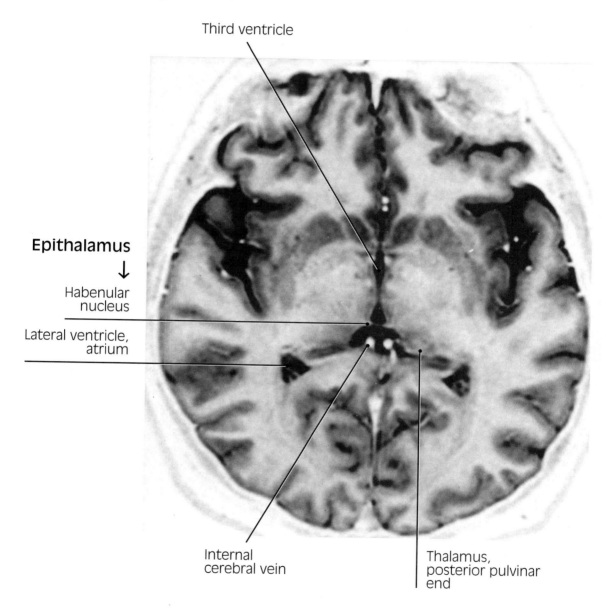

Third ventricle

**Epithalamus**
↓
Habenular
nucleus

Lateral ventricle,
atrium

Internal
cerebral vein

Thalamus,
posterior pulvinar
end

## Pineal Body (Epiphysis Cerebri)

Shape:   A small conical organ

Location:   Downward and backward between the superior colliculi

Below the splenium of the corpus callosum

Parts:   Body: Conical shape, about 8 mm in a maximum dimension

Stalk or peduncle: Divides anteriorly into two laminae, separated by the pineal recess of the third ventricle

Contents of each lamina of the stalk:

- Superior: Habenular commissure
- Inferior: Posterior commissure

**PRACTICAL POINTS**

Pinealocytes synthesize melatonin and serotonin, which have a role in growth and development.

Lesions:   Males: Precocious puberty

Pineal tumors: If large, cause obstructive hydrocephalus

Figure **4.16**

Epithalamus, sagittal view, magnified.

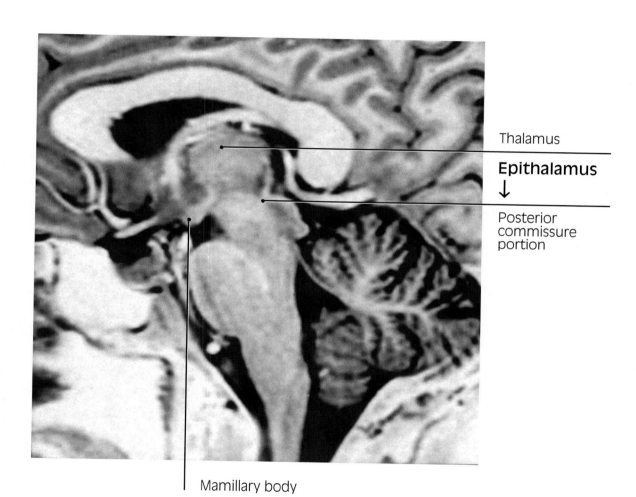

Thalamus

**Epithalamus**
↓

Posterior
commissure
portion

Mamillary body

Figure **4.17**

Epithalamus, sagittal view.

Thalamus

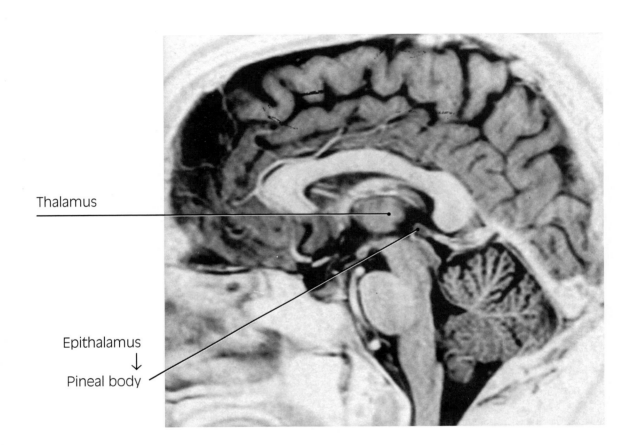

Epithalamus
↓
Pineal body

Figure **4.18**

Epithalamus, sagittal view, magnified.

Thalamus

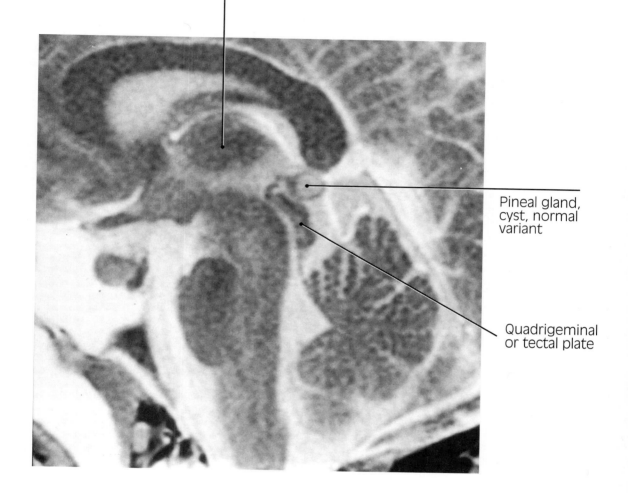

Pineal gland,
cyst, normal
variant

Quadrigeminal
or tectal plate

## Ventral Diencephalon

### Subthalamus

(Figures **4.19** to **4.21**)

Location:   Between the thalami above and the midbrain below

Medial to the internal capsule and the globus pallidus

Contents:   Gray matter:   Cranial ends of the red nucleus and substantia nigra

Subthalamic nucleus (body of Luys)

Zona incerta

White matter:   Cranial ends of lemnisci, lateral to the red nucleus

Dentothalamic tracts

Ansa ventricularis on the ventral surface

Fasciculus lenticularis on the dorsal surface

Subthalamic fasciculus

PRACTICAL POINT

**Lesions of the subthalamic nucleus:**   Hamiballismus

Figure **4.19**

Subthalamus, sagittal view.

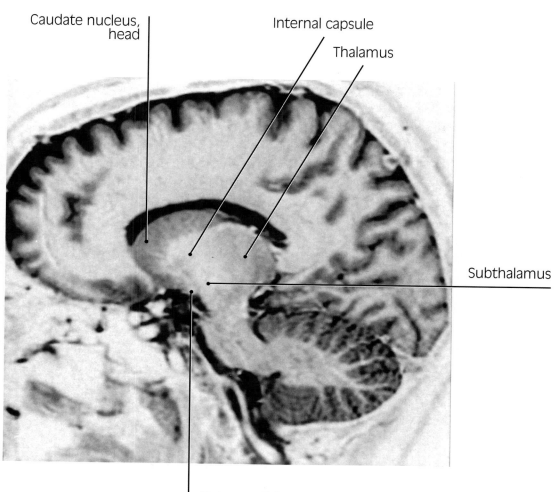

Caudate nucleus, head

Internal capsule

Thalamus

Subthalamus

Globus pallidus

Figure **4.20**

Subthalamus, sagittal view, magnified.

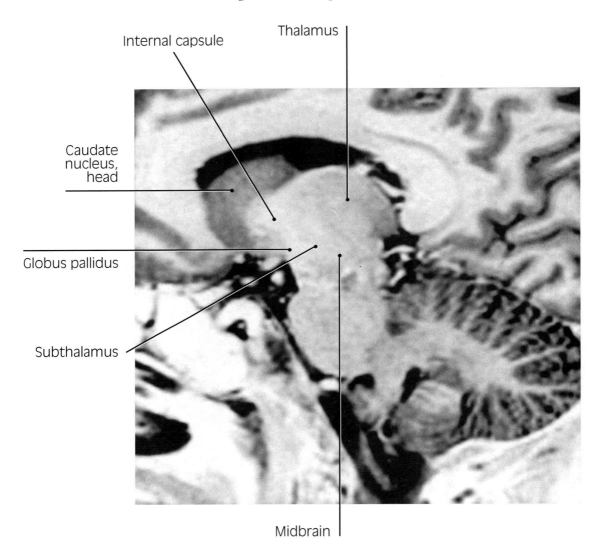

Internal capsule

Thalamus

Caudate
nucleus,
head

Globus pallidus

Subthalamus

Midbrain

Figure **4.21**

Metathalamus and subthalamus, axial view.

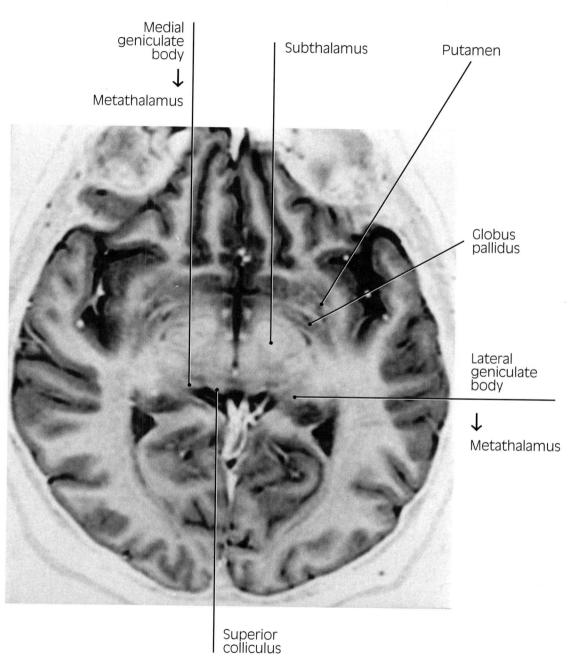

Medial
geniculate
body
↓
Metathalamus

Subthalamus

Putamen

Globus
pallidus

Lateral
geniculate
body
↓
Metathalamus

Superior
colliculus

## Hypothalamus
(Figures **4.22**, **4.23**, and **4.24**)

The hypothalamus is the inferior part of the diencephalon.

**Location:**  In the floor and lateral wall of the third ventricle

### Relationship When Viewed on the Base of the Brain

**Anterior:**  Optic chiasm

**Posterior:**  Posterior perforated substance

**Sides:**  Optic tract

Crus cerebri

### Relationship When Viewed in a Sagittal Section of the Brain

**Anterior:**  Lamina terminalis

**Posterior:**  Tegmentum of the midbrain

**Inferior:**  Floor of the third ventricle

**Posterosuperior:**  Hypothalamic sulcus

Figure **4.22**

Hypothalamus, sagittal view.

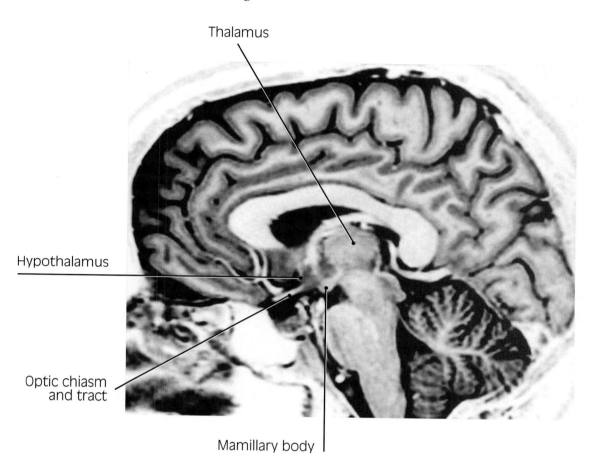

Thalamus

Hypothalamus

Optic chiasm
and tract

Mamillary body

Figure **4.23**

Hypothalamus, sagittal view, magnified.

Optic
tract

Hypothalamus

Thalamus, massa intermedia

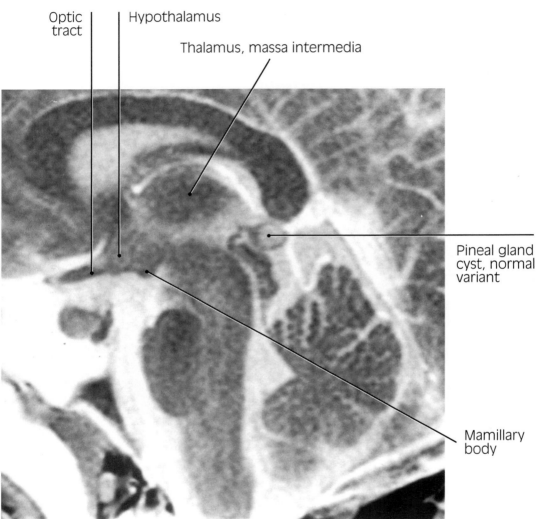

Pineal gland
cyst, normal
variant

Mamillary
body

Figure **4.24**

Thalamus, hypothalamus, and subthalamus, coronal view.

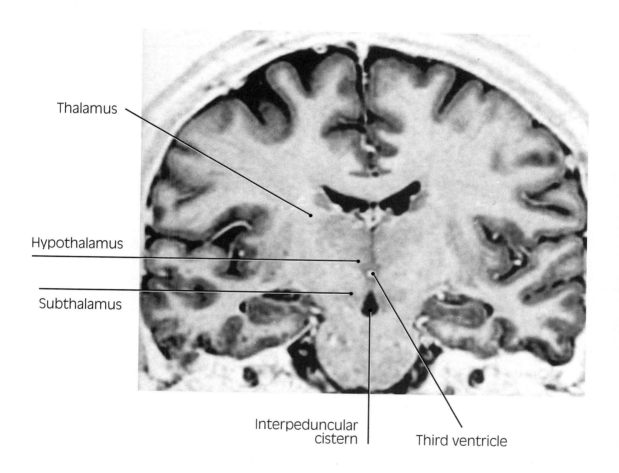

Thalamus

Hypothalamus

Subthalamus

Interpeduncular
cistern

Third ventricle

◻═══════════⬝ **Anatomic Divisions and Nuclei**

(Figure **4.25**)

| Divisions | Location | Nucleus (N) |
|-----------|----------|-------------|
| Optic | Rostral/anterior | Supraoptic N, above the optic chiasm<br>Paraventricular N, above the supraoptic nucleus |
| Tuberal | Intermediate | Ventromedial N<br>Dorsomedial N<br>Arcuate N<br>Tuberal or lateral N, lateral to ventromedial |
| Mamillary | Caudal/posterior | Posterior N, caudal to ventro- and dorsomedial N<br>Lateral N, lateral to posterior N |

## PRACTICAL POINTS

The hypothalamus is the head ganglion of the autonomic nervous system (ANS).

**Endocrine control:** Regulates secretion of releasing and release-inhibiting hormones: thyrotropin (TSH), corticotropin (ACTH), somatotropin (STH), prolactin, luteinizing hormone (LH), follicle-stimulating hormone (FSH), and melanocyte-stimulating hormone (MSH)

**Neurosecretion:** Oxytocin and vasopressin (antidiuretic hormone, ADH)

**General autonomic:** Parasympathetic by the anterior hypothalamus

Sympathetic by the posterior hypothalamus

**Temperature regulation:** Anterior hypothalamus: Rise in temperature

Posterior hypothalamus: Fall in temperature

**Food intakes:** Ventromedial nucleus: Inhibits hunger

Ventrolateral nucleus: Stimulates hunger

Sexual behavior and reproduction through its control on the anterior pituitary

Biological clocks such as sleep and wakefulness

Regulates emotion, fear, rage, aversion, pleasure, and reward (along with limbic system and the prefrontal cortex)

Figure **4.25**

Hypothalamus, sagittal view, magnified.

## Hypothalamus divisions

- Optic

- Tuberal

- Mamillary

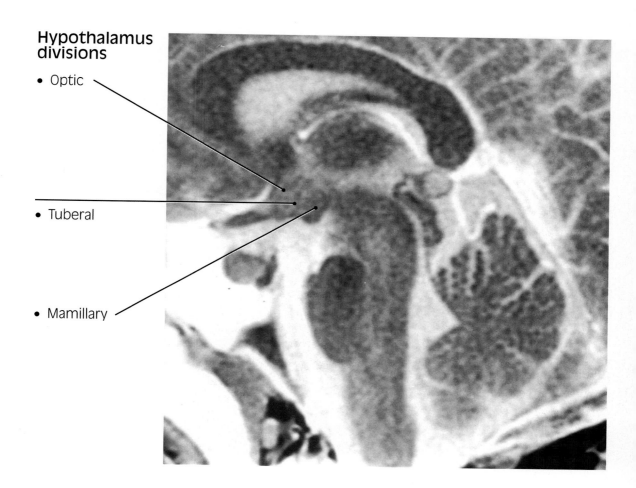

CHAPTER 5

# Limbic System or Rhinencephalon

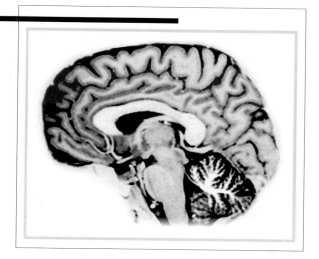

> The limbic system is a diverse group of medial and basal telencephalic structures with direct connection to the hypothalamus.

## Parts

An orbitofrontal cortex

Thalamic nuclei

Anterior perforated substance with the olfactory tubercle and the diagonal band of Broca

A limbic cortex

A piriform lobe with uncus

Hippocampal formation and fornix

Ammon's horn

Amygdala

Septum pellucidum with septal nuclei

Stria terminalis or stria habenularis

Anterior commissure

Mamillary bodies

## Orbitofrontal Cortex

(Figures **5.1** to **5.4**)

Olfactory nerves, bulb, and tract

Anterior olfactory nucleus

Medial, intermediate, and lateral olfactory striae

Medial and lateral olfactory gyri

Olfactory trigone

Figure **5.1**

Limbic system, orbitofrontal cortex, medial surface, sagittal view, magnified.

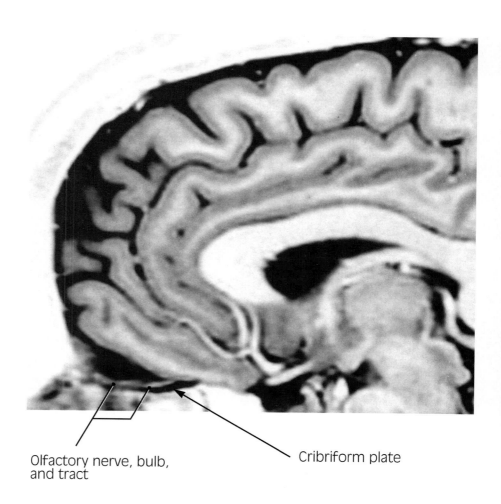

Olfactory nerve, bulb, and tract

Cribriform plate

PRACTICAL POINT

Mediates the conscious perception of smell

## Thalamic Nuclei

Medial dorsal and anterior

PRACTICAL POINTS

- The mediodorsal nucleus plays a role in behavior and memory.
- The anterior nucleus is a main link in the limbic circuit of Papez.

Figure **5.2**

Limbic system, olfactory cortex, sagittal view,
magnified.

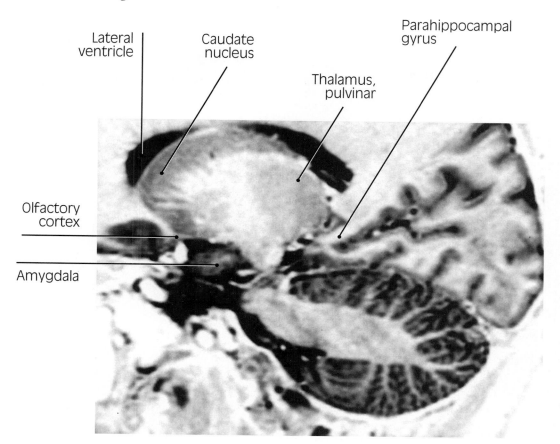

Figure **5.3**

Limbic system, orbitofrontal cortex, axial view.

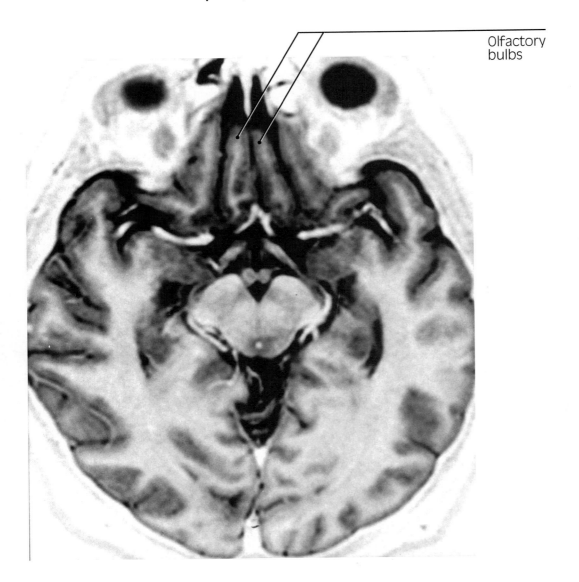

Olfactory
bulbs

Figure **5.4**

Limbic system, olfactory tract, coronal view.

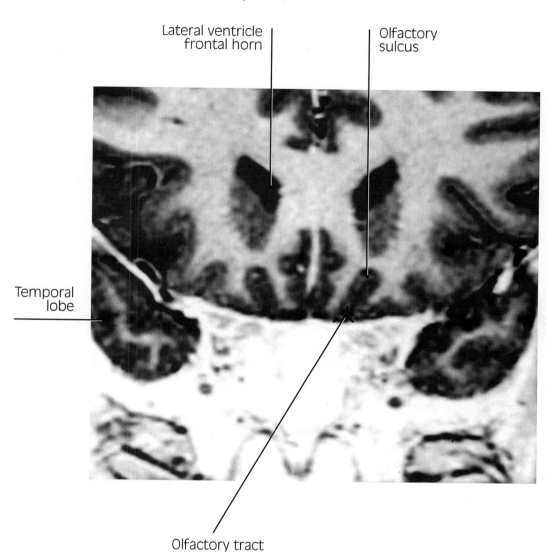

Lateral ventricle frontal horn

Olfactory sulcus

Temporal lobe

Olfactory tract

## Anterior Perforated Substance

(Figure **5.5**)

This is the important topographic landmark on the base of the brain.

**Location:**    Caudal to:  The olfactory trigone

The diverging medial and lateral olfactory striae

In the angle between: The optic chiasm and tract medially and the uncus laterally

**Relationships:**    Superior:  Corpus stratum and claustrum

Inferior:  Termination of the internal carotid artery

Origin of the anterior and middle cerebral arteries

Medial:  Tuber cinerium

Lateral:  Insula

A prepiriform cortex

Anterior:  Paraterminal gyrus

## Limbic Cortex

**Shape:**    C-shaped structure

**Location:**    Medial surface of the cerebral hemisphere, encircling the corpus callosum and lateral portion of the midbrain

**Parts:**    Paraolfactory gyrus or subcallosal area

Paraterminal gyrus

Anterior and posterior parts of the parahippocampal gyrus

Posterior part of the cingulate gyrus

An insular cortex

**Contents:**    Hippocampal formation

Amygdaloid nuclear complex

Figure **5.5**

Limbic system, anterior perforated substance,
sagittal view, magnified.

Fornix

Mamillary
body

Anterior
perforated
substance

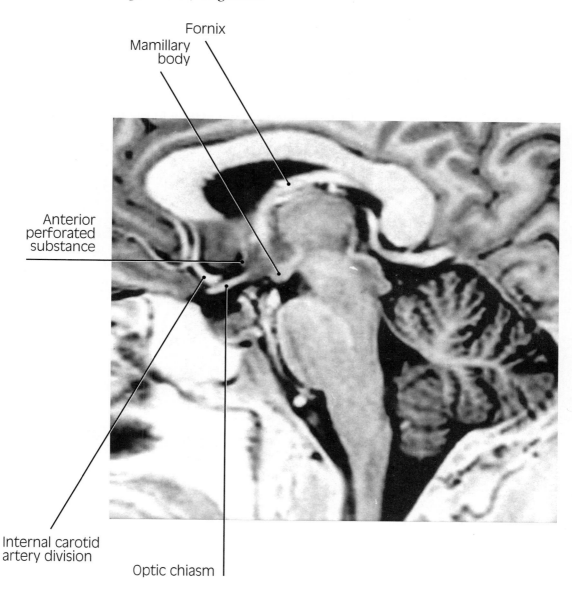

Internal carotid
artery division

Optic chiasm

### Paraolfactory Gyrus or Subcallosal Area

(Figure 5.6)

Location:  Between the anterior and posterior paraolfactory sulci

In front of the lamina terminalis

Ventral to the rostrum of the corpus callosum

### Paraterminal Gyrus

Location:  A narrow triangular fold of gray matter in front of the lamina terminalis and ventral to the rostrum of the corpus callosum

### Parahippocampal Gyrus

(Figures 5.7 and 5.8)

Most medial convolution of the temporal lobe

Location:  Between the hippocampal and collateral sulci

Contents:  Entorhinal areas

Subicular areas

Termination:  In the uncus

Figure **5.6**

Limbic system, paraolfactory gyrus or subcallosal area, sagittal view, magnified.

Corpus callosum

Anterior commissure

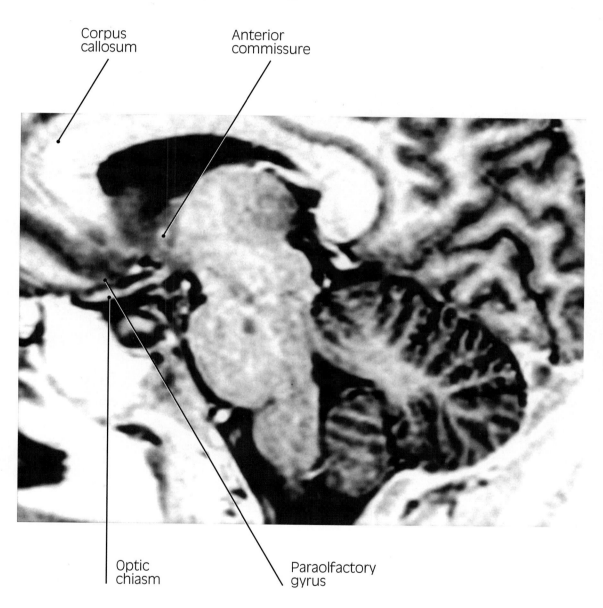

Optic chiasm

Paraolfactory gyrus

Figure **5.7**

Limbic system, parahippocampus, sagittal view,
magnified.

Parahippocampal gyrus

Cerebral peduncle

Cingulum and
cingulate gyrus

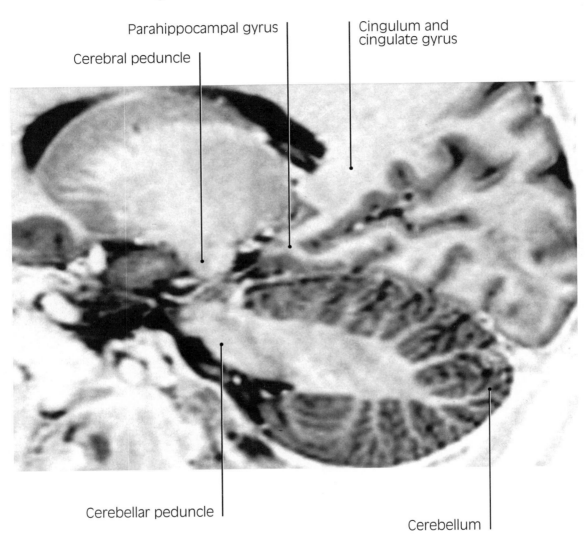

Cerebellar peduncle

Cerebellum

Figure **5.8**

Limbic system, parahippocampus, sagittal view.

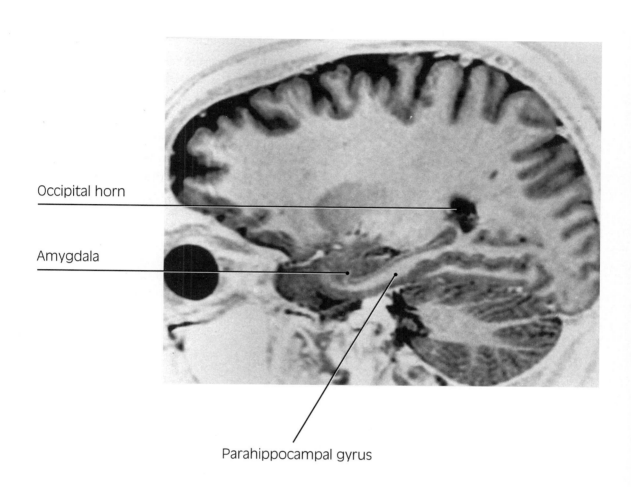

Occipital horn

Amygdala

Parahippocampal gyrus

## Cingulate Gyrus

(Figures **5.9** to **5.11**)

**Shape:** The horseshoe-shaped cortical strip

**Location:** Long gyrus above the corpus callosum

**Origin:** Below the rostrum of the corpus callosum

**Course:** Follows the corpus callosum and is separated by the collateral sulcus

**Termination:** Merges with the parahippocampal gyrus at the isthmus after coursing round the inferior surface of the splenium of the corpus callosum

**Cingulum:** A bundle of association fibers that runs in the white core of the cingulate and the parahippocampal gyri

**PRACTICAL POINT**

A lesion of the cingulate gyrus results in akinesia, mutism, and apathy.

Figure **5.9**

Limbic system, cingulate gyrus, fornix, anterior commissure, and mamillary body, sagittal view.

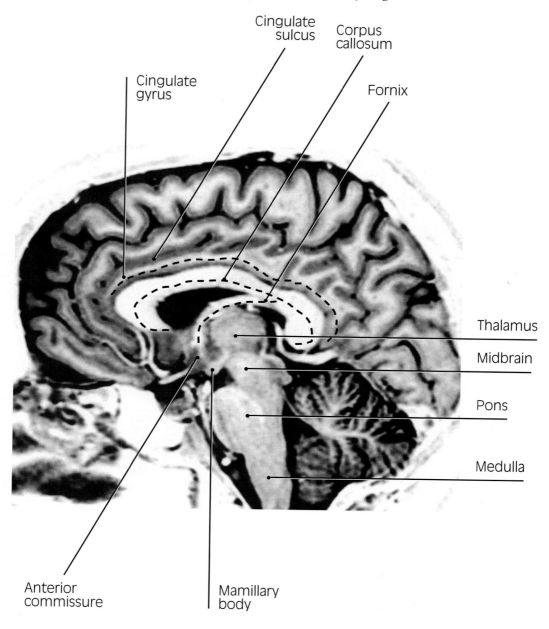

Cingulate sulcus

Corpus callosum

Cingulate gyrus

Fornix

Thalamus

Midbrain

Pons

Medulla

Anterior commissure

Mamillary body

Figure **5.10**

Limbic system, cingulate gyrus and fornix, axial view.

Cingulate
gyrus

Fornix

Cingulate
gyrus

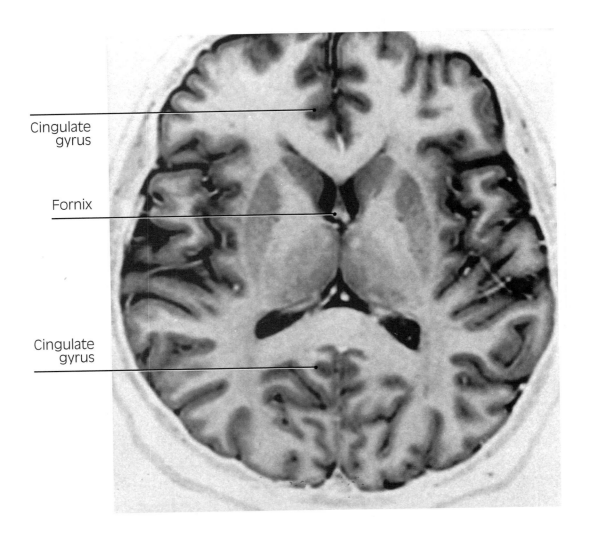

Figure **5.11**

Limbic system, cingulate gyrus, septum pellucidum, amygdala, coronal view.

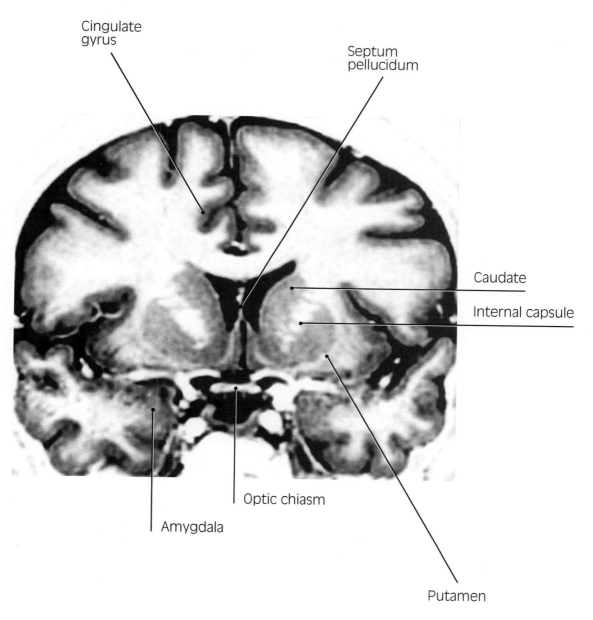

Cingulate gyrus

Septum pellucidum

Caudate

Internal capsule

Optic chiasm

Amygdala

Putamen

## Insular Cortex

(Figure **5.12**)

Location:    Deep in the floor of the lateral sulcus and surrounded
by the circular sulcus

Parts:    Cortical areas or the opercula of the insula

Separated by the ascending and posterior rami of the lateral
sulcus

### Frontal Operculum

Formation:    By the pars triangularis of the inferior frontal gyrus

Location:    Between the ascending and the anterior rami

### Frontoparietal Operculum

Formation:    By the pars posterior of the inferior frontal gyrus

Lower ends of the pre- and postcentral gyri

Lower anterior part of the inferior parietal lobule

Location:    Between the ascending and upturned turn of the
posterior ramus of the lateral sulcus

### Temporal Operculum

Formation:    By the superior temporal and transverse temporal gyri

Location:    Below the posterior ramus of the lateral sulcus

### Apex of the Insula or Limen Insulae or Gyrus Ambiens

Divisions:    By the sulcus centralis insulae

Parts:    Anterior three to four short gyri

Posterior long gyrus

## Piriform Lobe

Part of the olfactory system

Contents:    Lateral olfactory gyrus

Lateral olfactory stria

Uncus hippocampi

Entorhinal or cranial part of the parahippocampal gyrus

Figure **5.12**

Limbic system, insula, axial view, magnified.

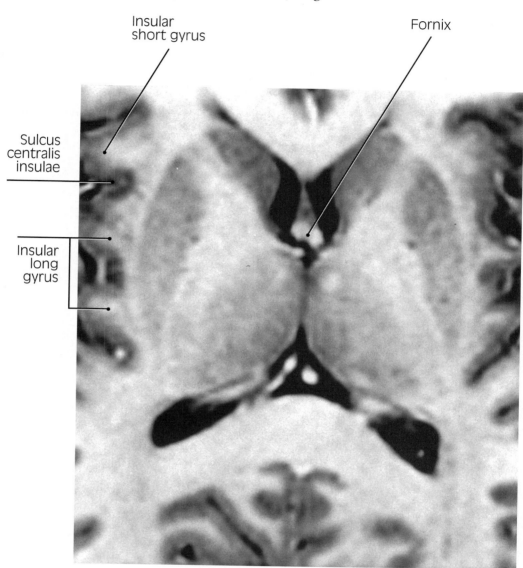

Insular
short gyrus

Fornix

Sulcus
centralis
insulae

Insular
long
gyrus

## The Uncus

(Figure **5.13**)

**Shape:**   Hooklike

**Location:**   At the anterior end of the parahippocampal gyrus and forms the posterolateral boundary of the anterior perforated substance

**Contents:**   Uncinate gyrus

Tail of the dentate gyrus or band of Giacomini

Intralimbic gyrus

Figure **5.13**

Limbic system, uncus, coronal view.

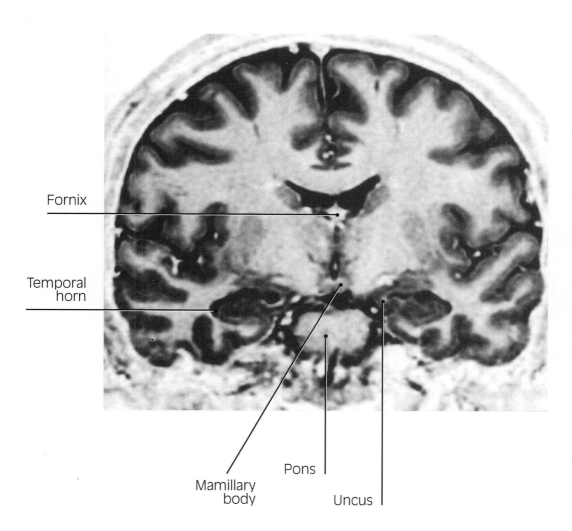

## Hippocampal Formation

(Figures **5.14** and **5.15**)

The most important feature of the medial temporal lobe

**Embryology:**   Develops in the medial pallial fringe of the cerebral hemisphere, immediately next to the outer convex border of the choroidal fissure

**Location:**   Along the floor of the inferior horn of the lateral ventricle, below the corpus callosum

**Components:**   Prehippocampal rudiments

Gray matter: Dentate gyrus

Subiculum

Ammon's horn:  Cornu Ammonis

Hippocampus

White matter: Alveus

Fimbria

Fornix

The gray and white matter structures are arranged around the corpus callosum, the hippocampal fissure, and the callosal sulcus.

Figure **5.14**

Limbic system, hippocampus and parahippocampus, sagittal view, magnified.

Subiculum   Hippocampal        Alveus
              fissure

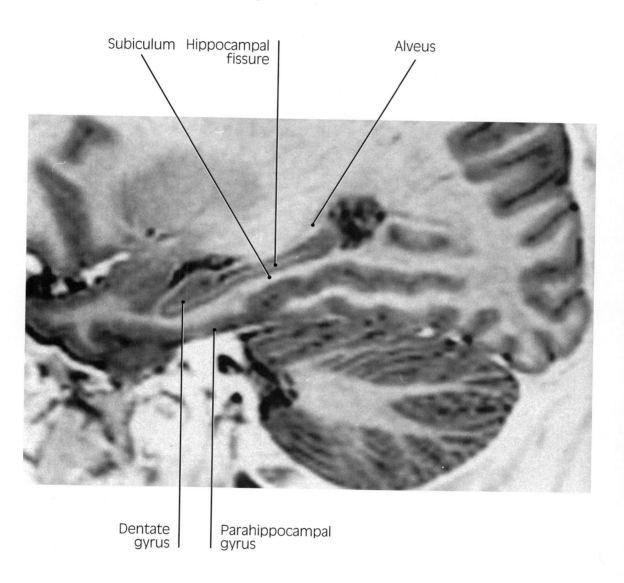

Dentate   Parahippocampal
gyrus     gyrus

## Hippocampal Fissure

A horizontal fissure that lies immediately above the parahippocampal gyrus. It extends the full length of the temporal lobe and then continues around and behind the splenium to become the callosal sulcus.

## Prehippocampal Rudiments

Contents:   Indusium griseum

Gyrus fasciolaris

Longitudinal striae

Figure **5.15**

Limbic system, hippocampus and uncus, coronal view, magnified.

Temporal horn

Hippocampal sulcus

Uncus

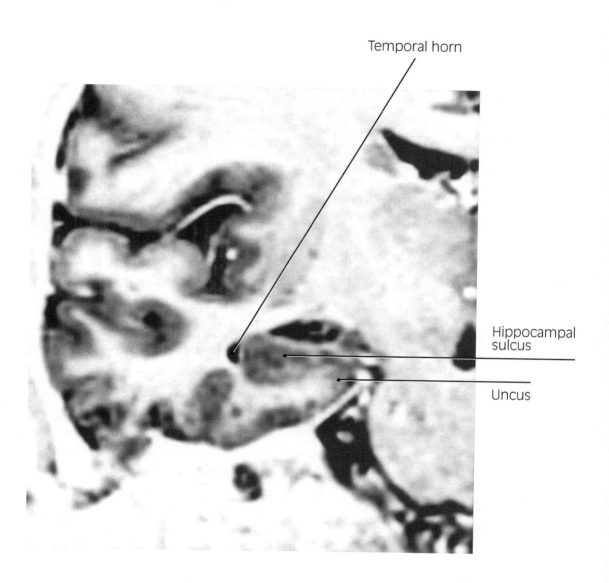

## Indusium Griseum or Supracallosal Gyrus

(Figures **5.16** and **5.17**)

Location: A thin veil of gray matter covering the superior surface of the corpus callosum

Course: Passes into the callosal sulcus and continuous with the cortex of the cingulate gyrus from the rostrum of the corpus callosum to the splenium. It then diverges to become the right and the left gyrus fasciolaris or the splenial gyri.

> **N O T E** The medial and lateral longitudinal striae of Lancisi are two narrow bundles of the white fibers embedded in the indusium.

## Dentate Gyrus

Forms the upper bank of the hippocampal fissure

Appearance: Dentate or crenated because of multiple transverse grooves in a narrow cortical band

Relationships: Superior: Recurved part of the cornu Ammonis alveus

Inferior: Subiculum

Medial: Fimbria of the fornix

Lateral: Cornu Ammonis

Anterior: Continued into the uncus notch

Posterior: Smooth and featureless tail of the dentate gyrus, or band of Giacomini

(Figures **5.18** to **5.20**)

## Subiculum

Forms the lower bank of the hippocampal fissure

> **N O T E** Histologically, at the beginning of the Ammon's horn, it exhibits a four-layered type of cortex instead of a modified six-layered cortex.

Figure **5.16**

Limbic system, prehippocampal rudiments,
coronal view.

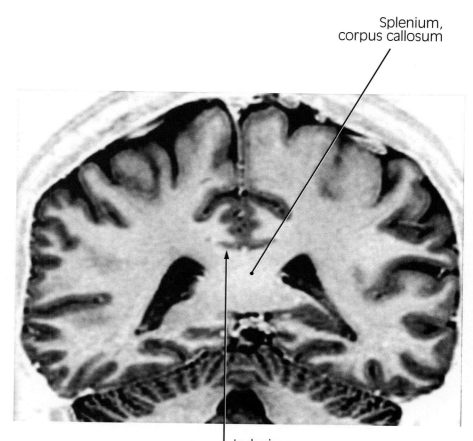

Splenium,
corpus callosum

Indusium
griseum

Figure **5.17**

Limbic system, indusium griseum, fornix, mamillary body, coronal view.

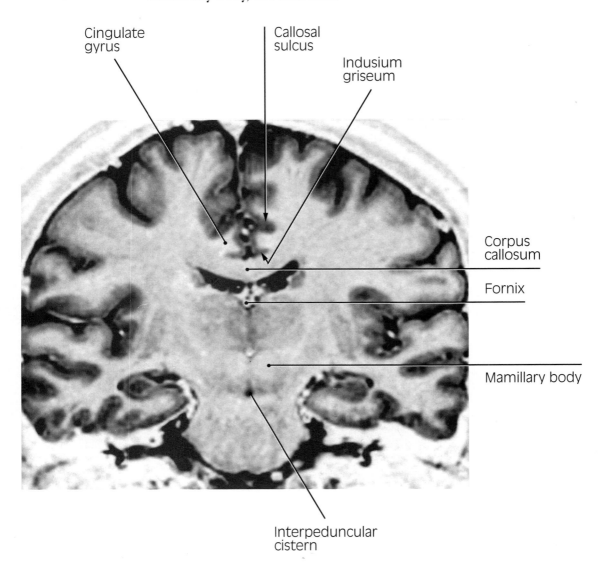

Cingulate gyrus

Callosal sulcus

Indusium griseum

Corpus callosum

Fornix

Mamillary body

Interpeduncular cistern

Figure **5.18**

Limbic system, hippocampus and parahippocampus, coronal view, magnified.

Alveus

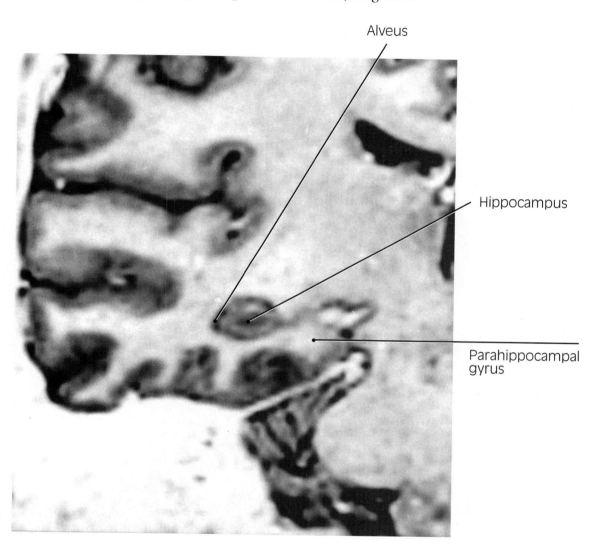

Hippocampus

Parahippocampal gyrus

Figure **5.19**

Limbic system, hippocampus and parahippocampus, coronal view, magnified.

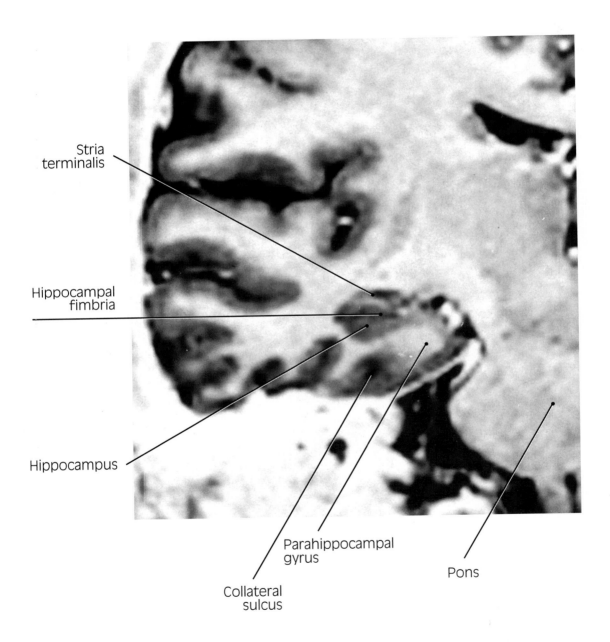

Stria terminalis

Hippocampal fimbria

Hippocampus

Parahippocampal gyrus

Collateral sulcus

Pons

Figure **5.20**

Limbic system, hippocampus, coronal view, magnified.

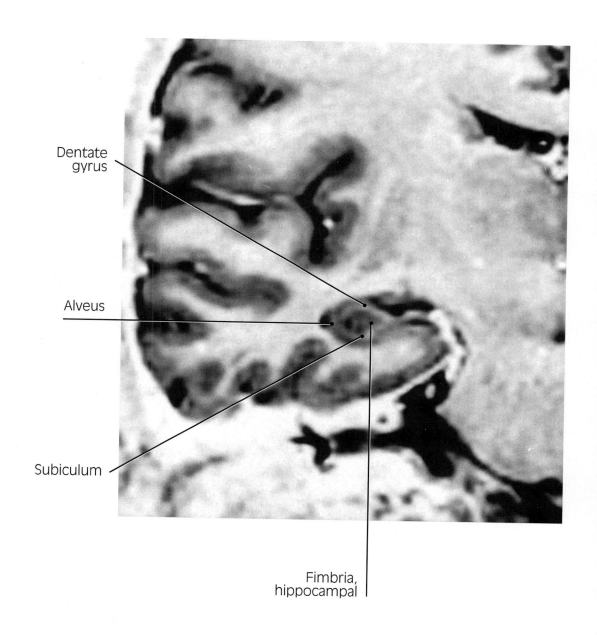

Dentate
gyrus

Alveus

Subiculum

Fimbria,
hippocampal

**Location:** Along the superior surface of the parahippocampal gyrus

**Zones:** Parasubiculum

Presubiculum

Subiculum

Prosubiculum

# Ammon's Horn

(Figure **5.21**)

A cytoarchitectural pattern is roughly similar throughout the Ammon's horn.

We subdivide this region into a series of radially disposed fields that do not correspond to each other:

- Cornu Ammonis (CA) Fields: CA1 to CA4 of Lorente de No

- Hippocampal (H) Fields: H1 to H5 of Rose

## Alveus

A thin subependymal sheet of white matter that covers the lateral surface of the hippocampus, separating it from the ependyma of the temporal horn. Its medial free margin (of white matter) is called the fimbria of the fornix.

Figure **5.21**

Limbic system, hippocampus, coronal view, magnified.

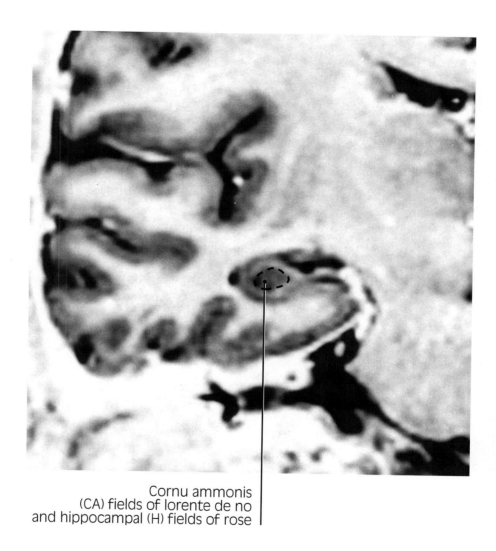

Cornu ammonis
(CA) fields of lorente de no
and hippocampal (H) fields of rose

## Fornix

(Figure **5.22**)

**Shape:**   Long C-shaped bundle of white matter

**Parts:**   Alveus

Fimbria

Crus

Body

Column

**Alveus:**   As discussed above

**Fimbria:**   A flattened band of white fibers at the medial free margin of the alveus, which lies superior to the dentate gyrus and forms the inferior boundary of the choroidal fissure. It extends the length of the hippocampal formation above the hippocampal fissure.

**Crus:**   This is the superior arch of the fimbria, anterior and inferior to the splenium. The crura are closely applied to the inferior surface of the corpus callosum and form the anterior inferior medial walls of the atrium. The crura are interconnected to each other by the transverse fibers that pass between the hippocampal formation of two sides and form the commissure of the fornix or hippocampal commissure. The commissure is a thin triangular sheet and is seen beneath the body of the corpus callosum.

**Body:**   The anterior midline fusion of the crura is the body of the fornix. It lies above the tela choroidea and the ependymal roof of the third ventricle. It is attached to the inferior surface of the corpus callosum and more anteriorly to the inferior borders of the laminae of the septum pellucidum.

**Column:**   Anteriorly, above the interventricular foramina, the body of the fornix diverges into the right and the left bundles, or the columns. They curve inferiorly toward the anterior commissure, forming the anterior boundary of the foramina. Each column continues to curve inferoposteriorly and gradually sinks into the corresponding part of the lateral wall of the third ventricle to reach the superior aspect of the mamillary body.

**Choroidal fissure:**   A cleft between the lateral edge of the fornix (or taenia fornicis) and a small ridge of tissue that encircles the diencephalon (or taenia choroidea). The latter invaginates into the ventricle through the choroidal fissure to form the choroid plexus.

Figure **5.22**

Limbic system, fornix and anterior commissure, sagittal view, magnified.

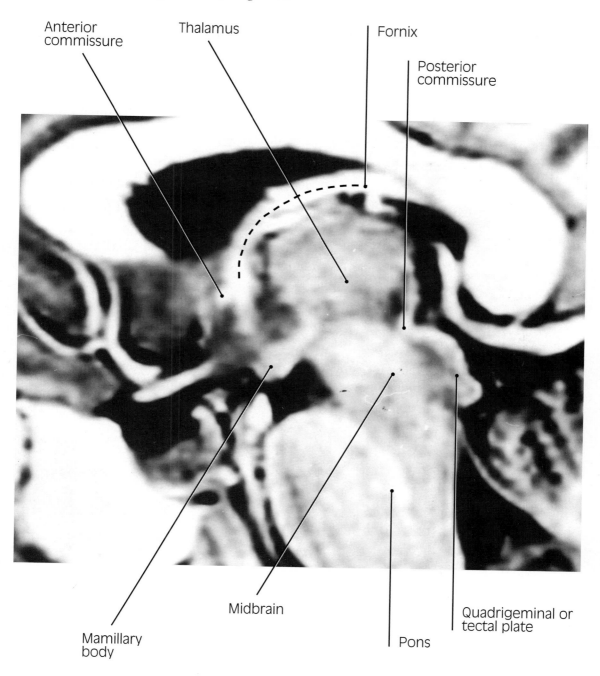

Anterior
commissure

Thalamus

Fornix

Posterior
commissure

Mamillary
body

Midbrain

Pons

Quadrigeminal or
tectal plate

The hippocampus is involved in learning and memory, mainly long-term memories.

## Amygdala

(Figures **5.23** and **5.24**)

**Shape:**   Resembles that of an almond

**Location:**   Large nuclear complex forming the anterior wall of the temporal lobe, underlying the parahippocampal uncus

**Histology:**   Same tissue as the basal ganglia

**Relationships:**   Superior: Continues with claustrum

Also related to the external capsule

Caudal: Closely related to the ventral part of the hippocampus

Fuses with the tip of the tail of the caudate nucleus

**Nuclei:**   Corticomedial

Basilateral

Lesions of the amygdaloid complex result in placidity, with loss of fear, rage, aggression, and hypersexual behavior.

Figure **5.23**

Limbic system, amygdala and mamillary body, axial view.

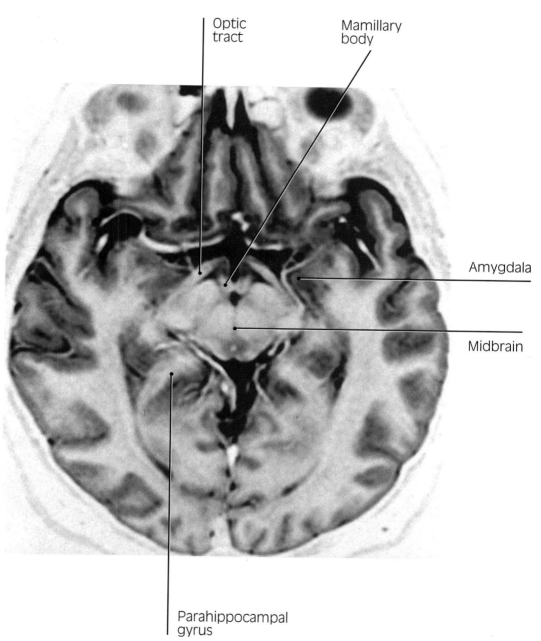

Optic tract

Mamillary body

Amygdala

Midbrain

Parahippocampal gyrus

## Septal Nuclei

The septal areas or nuclei are the nuclear masses of gray matter at the medial walls of the cerebral hemispheres. They are situated immediately anterior and superior to the lamina terminalis and the anterior commissure.

## Septum Pellucidum

Location: Midline of the cerebrum, anterior and superior to the hypothalamus

### PRACTICAL CONSIDERATION

In control of temper and the autonomic system

## Stria Terminalis or Stria Semicircularis

A long bundle of fibers that lies in the groove that separates the thalamus and the caudate nucleus. It courses posteriorly along the striothalamic groove in the floor of the lateral ventricle, close to the thalamostriate vein. It ends in the amygdala after its course around the atrium and the tail of the caudate nucleus.

Figure **5.24**

Limbic system, amygdala, sagittal view.

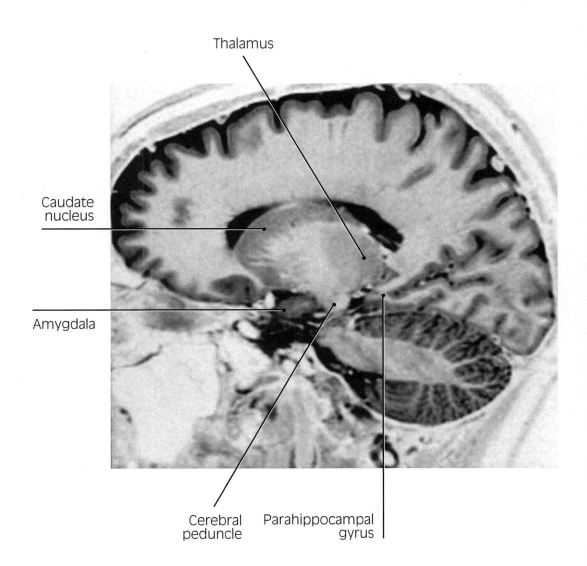

Thalamus

Caudate
nucleus

Amygdala

Cerebral
peduncle

Parahippocampal
gyrus

## Anterior Commissure

(Figure **5.25**)

A compact bundle of white fibers that crosses the midline in the lamina terminalis just under the rostrum of the corpus callosum

## Mamillary Bodies

(Figure **5.26**)

Location:    Posterior to hypothalamus

### PRACTICAL POINT

They decide mood and the degree of wakefulness.

Figure **5.25**

Limbic system, anterior commissure and septum pellucidum, coronal view.

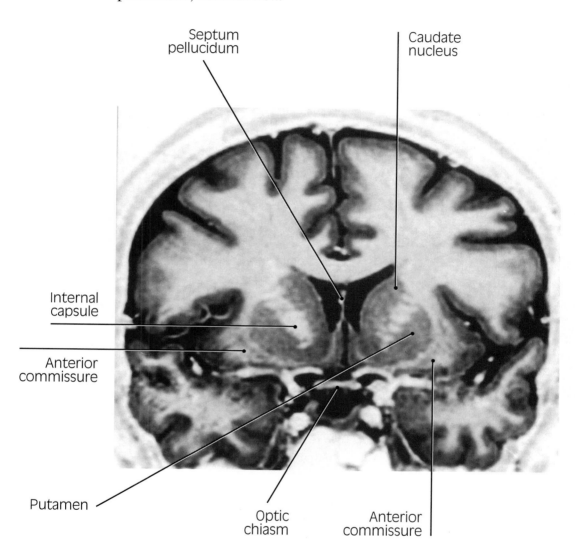

Septum pellucidum

Caudate nucleus

Internal capsule

Anterior commissure

Putamen

Optic chiasm

Anterior commissure

Figure **5.26**

Limbic system, mamillary body and amygdala, axial view, magnified.

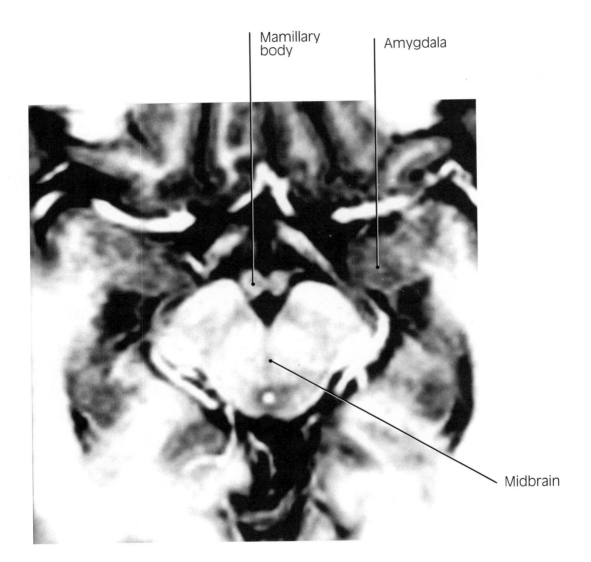

Mamillary body

Amygdala

Midbrain

CHAPTER *6*

# Pituitary Gland

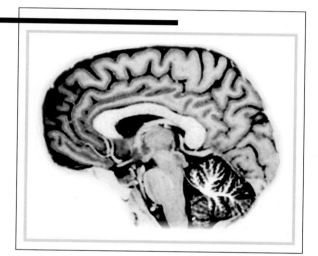

143

> "The leader of the endocrine orchestra," the pituitary produces most of the hormones that control the functions of many other endocrine glands in the body.

(Figures **6.1** to **6.8**)

## Location

In the hypophyseal or pituitary fossa or sella turcica

## Relationships

Superior:  Diaphragmatic sella

Optic chiasm

Tuber cinereum

Infundibular recess of the third ventricle

Inferior:  Venous sinuses in the dura of the sellar floor

Bony sella

Sphenoid sinus

Either side:  Cavernous sinuses and their contents

Internal carotid arteries and the sixth cranial nerves

## Divisions

Anterior lobe or adenohypophysis

Posterior lobe or neurohypophysis

### Adenohypophysis

A true endocrine organ

Origin:  Ectodermal

From the superior invagination of Ratke's pouch from the fetal nasopharynx

MRI characteristics:  Isointense to gray matter on unenhanced T1-weighted images

Figure **6.1**

Pituitary gland, sagittal view, magnified.

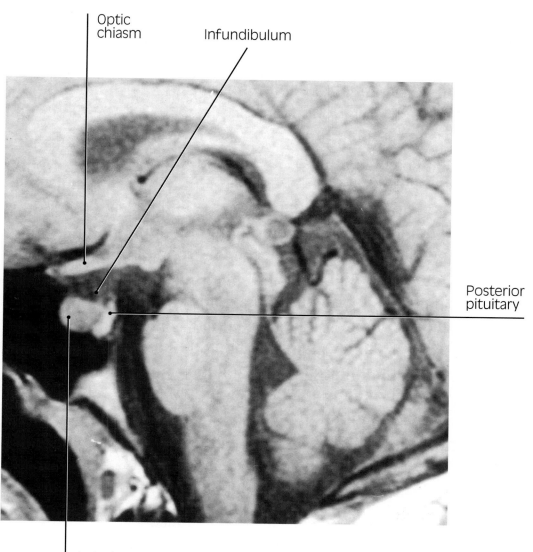

Optic chiasm

Infundibulum

Posterior pituitary

Anterior pituitary

Subdivisions: Anterior lobe: Pars anterior, the largest of all
Pars distalis
Pars glandularis

Pars distalis: forms most of the intrasellar adenohypophysis

Intermediate lobe, or pars intermedia:

Intraglandular cleft or a remnant of the lumen of Rathke's pouch

Vestigial, no physiologic purpose, may be the site of nonfunctioning cysts

Tuberal part, or pars tuberalis: An upward extension of the anterior lobe that surrounds and forms part of the infundibulum

# Neurohypophysis

**Origin:** From the hypothalamus as a downward growth into the sella

**MRI characteristics:** Hyperintense on T1-weighted images

Less hyperintense on T2-weighted images

**Divisions:** Posterior or neural lobe or pars posterior

Pituitary or infundibular stalk or hypothalamohypophyseal tract—the central landmark, wide superiorly and tapers inferiorly

Median eminence of the tuber cinereum

Paraventricular and supraoptic hypothalamic nuclei

**PRACTICAL POINTS**

Hormones are mediated via the hypothalamohypophyseal tract

### Pituitary Hormones

| Anterior | Posterior |
|---|---|
| Corticotropin | Antidiuretic hormone |
| Growth hormone | Oxytocin |
| Follicle stimulating hormone | |
| Luteinizing hormone | |
| Thyroid-stimulating hormone | |
| Prolactin | |

Figure **6.2**

Pituitary gland, sagittal view, magnified.

Anterior
pituitary

Infundibular
stalk

Posterior
pituitary

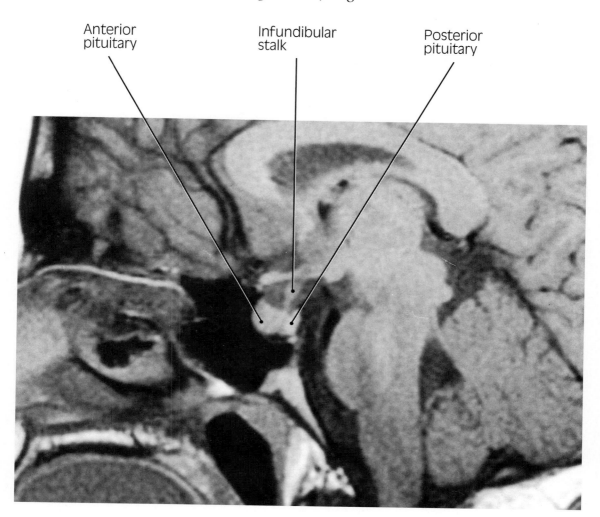

> **N O T E**   Absence of high signal of the posterior pituitary may be associated with central diabetes insipidus or suggestive of compressive lesions of the pituitary gland.

## Suprasellar Cisterns

Critical space

**Shape:**   Six-pointed star on axial images

**Net formed by:**   Anterior: Interhemispheric fissure

Anterolateral: Paired sylvian cisterns

Posterolateral: Paired ambient cisterns

Posterior: Interpeduncular cistern

**Contents:**   Cranial nerves III, IV, V1 and V2, and VI

Optic chiasm

Vascular anastomoses of the circle of Willis

Inferior hypothalamus

Pituitary infundibulum with its venous plexus

Figure **6.3**

Pituitary gland, sagittal view, magnified.

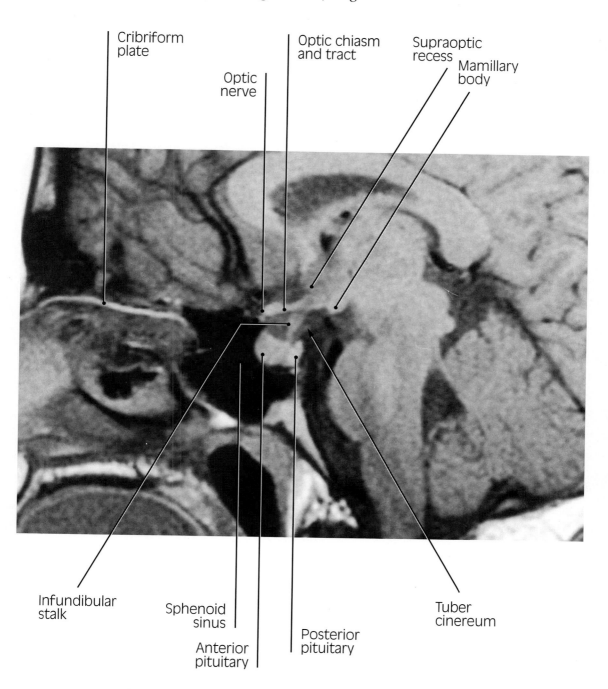

Figure **6.4**

Pituitary gland, coronal view.

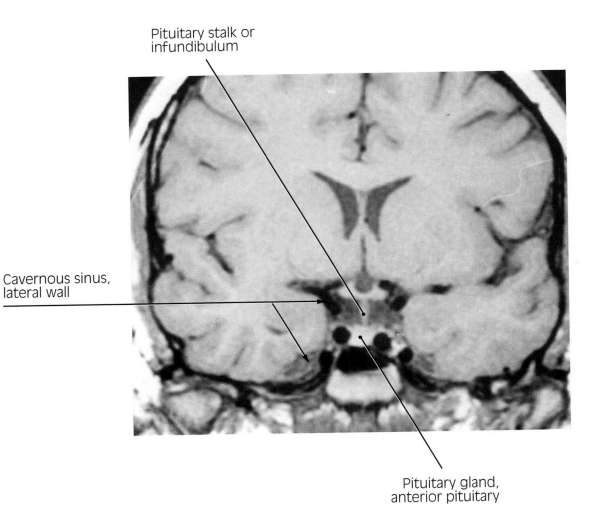

Pituitary stalk or
infundibulum

Cavernous sinus,
lateral wall

Pituitary gland,
anterior pituitary

Figure **6.5**

Pituitary gland, coronal view, magnified.

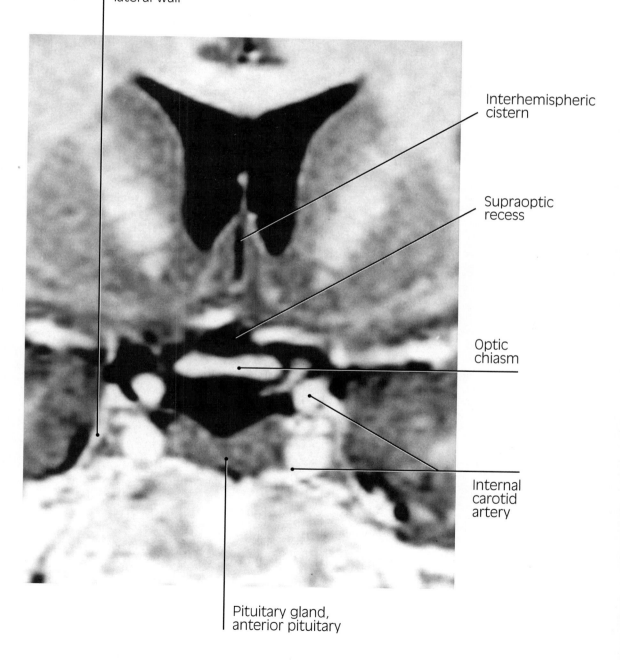

Cavernous sinus,
lateral wall

Interhemispheric
cistern

Supraoptic
recess

Optic
chiasm

Internal
carotid
artery

Pituitary gland,
anterior pituitary

Figure **6.6**

Pituitary gland, coronal view, magnified.

Infundibulum

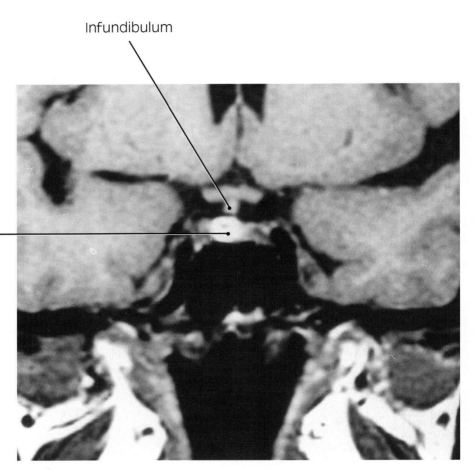

Pituitary gland,
posterior
pituitary
(bright signal,
normal variant)

Figure **6.7**

Pituitary gland, coronal view.

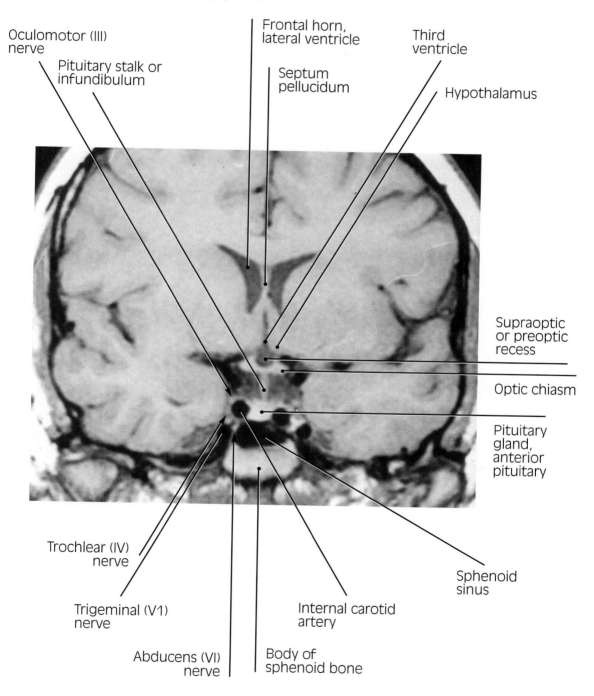

Oculomotor (III) nerve

Pituitary stalk or infundibulum

Frontal horn, lateral ventricle

Septum pellucidum

Third ventricle

Hypothalamus

Supraoptic or preoptic recess

Optic chiasm

Pituitary gland, anterior pituitary

Trochlear (IV) nerve

Trigeminal (V1) nerve

Abducens (VI) nerve

Internal carotid artery

Body of sphenoid bone

Sphenoid sinus

Figure **6.8**

Pituitary gland, coronal view, magnified.

Infundibulum

Optic chiasm

Oculomotor
(III) nerve

Trochlear
(IV) nerve

Trigeminal
(V1) nerve

Abducens
(VI) nerve

Pituitary
gland

Internal
carotid artery

Trigeminal (V2)
nerve

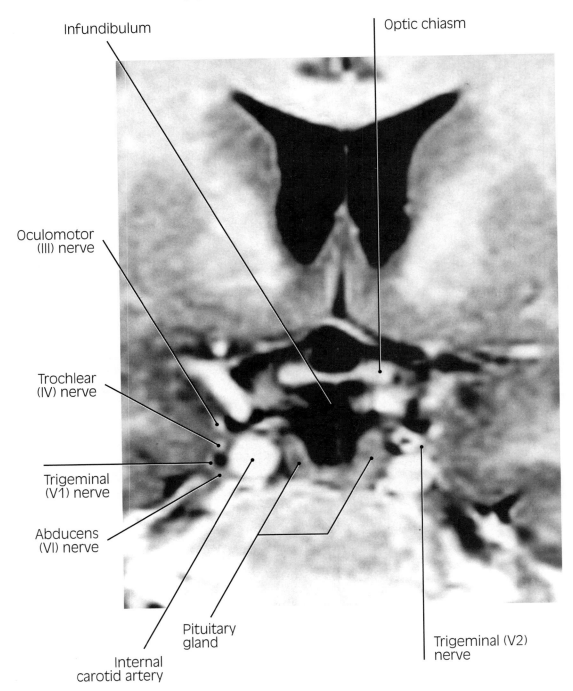

CHAPTER 7

# Mesencephalon
# or Midbrain

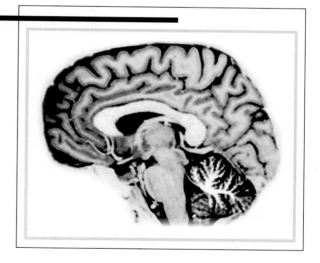

> The midbrain connects the diencephalon to the hindbrain. Its cavity, the cerebral aqueduct or aqueduct of Sylvius, connects the third with the fourth ventricle.

## FUNCTIONAL CONSIDERATION

The narrow diameter of the cerebral aqueduct makes it a frequent site for obstruction to the flow of cerebrospinal fluid.

## Relationships

Anterior:    Interpeduncular structures

Posterior:    Splenium of the corpus callosum

Great cerebral vein

Pineal body

Posterior ends of the thalami

Either side:    Parahippocampal gyri

Optic tracts

Posterior cerebral artery

Basal vein

Geniculate bodies

## Parts

(Figures **7.1** to **7.5**)

### Anterior

Midline:    Interpeduncular fossa, seen as a deep notch

Either side:    Crus cerebri

Oculomotor nerve:    Between the interpeduncular fossa and the crus cerebri

### Posterior

Corpora quadrigemina, seen as four rounded swellings

Superior and inferior colliculi

Trochlear nerve below the inferior colliculi in the midline

Figure **7.1**

Midbrain, sagittal view, magnified.

Thalamus   Midbrain or
mesencephalon   Vein of
Galen

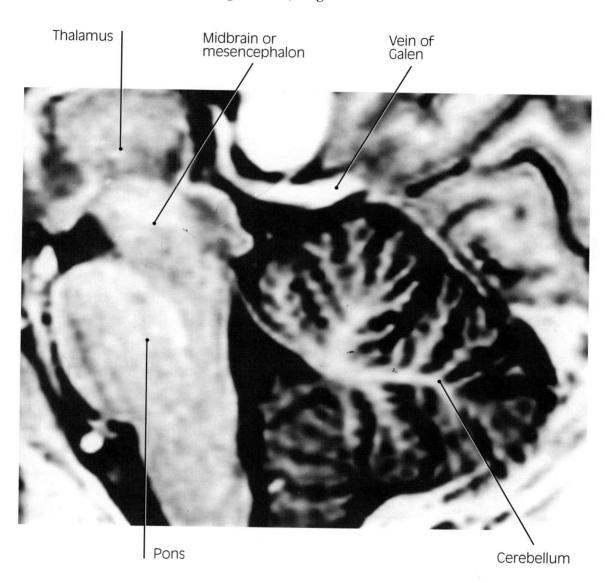

Pons   Cerebellum

## Divisions

### The Tectum

The part posterior to the aqueduct, made up of the right and left superior and inferior colliculi

### Cerebral Peduncle

We know that each half of the midbrain anterior to the aqueduct is the cerebral peduncle.

**Subdivisions:** Anterior: Crus cerebri

Middle: Substantia nigra

Posterior: Tegmentum

Figure **7.2**

Midbrain (tectal plate), sagittal view, magnified.

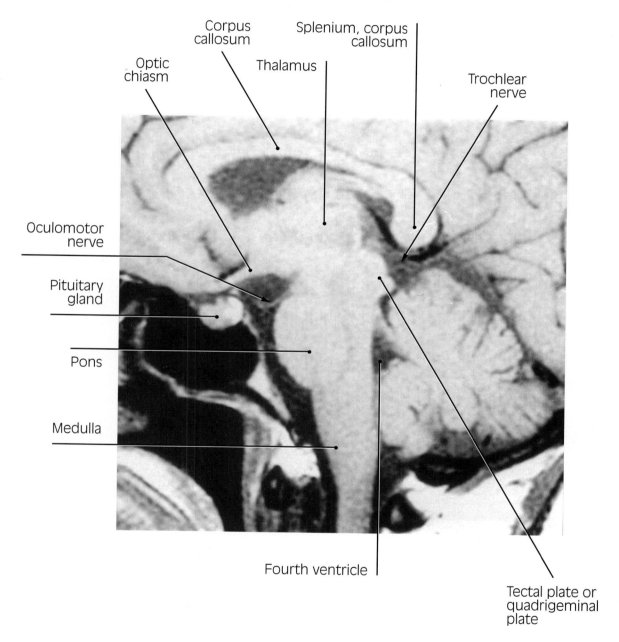

> **N O T E** The substantia nigra separates the crus cerebri and the tegmentum, and they form the cerebral peduncle.

Connections: Superior colliculus to the lateral geniculate body by the superior brachium

Inferior colliculus to the medial geniculate body by the inferior brachium

Figure **7.3**

Midbrain (parts), sagittal view, magnified.

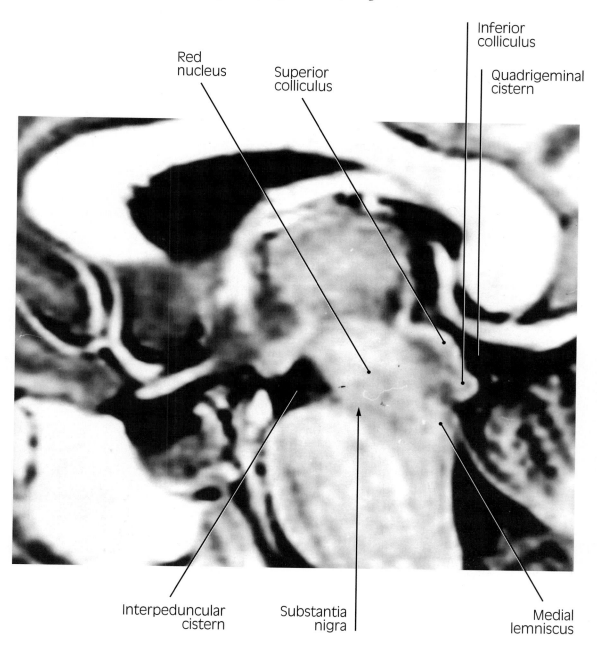

Figure **7.4**

Midbrain, corpora quadrigemina, sagittal view,
magnified (quadrigeminal or tectal plate).

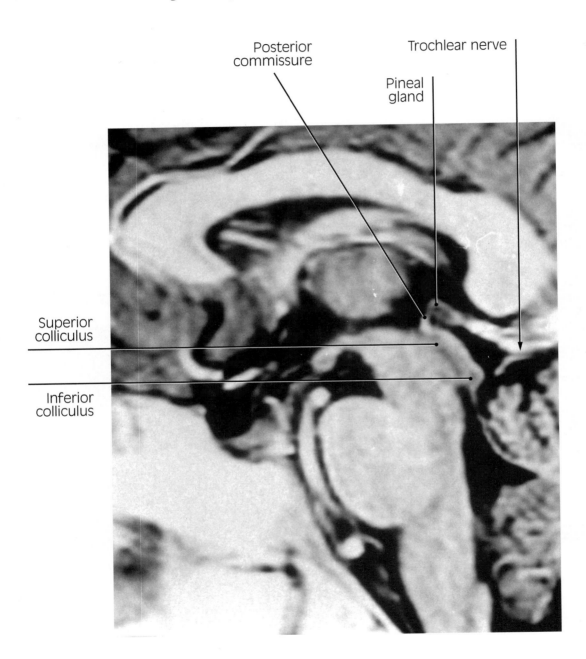

Figure **7.5**

Midbrain, corpora quadrigemina, coronal view,
(quadrigeminal or tectal plate).

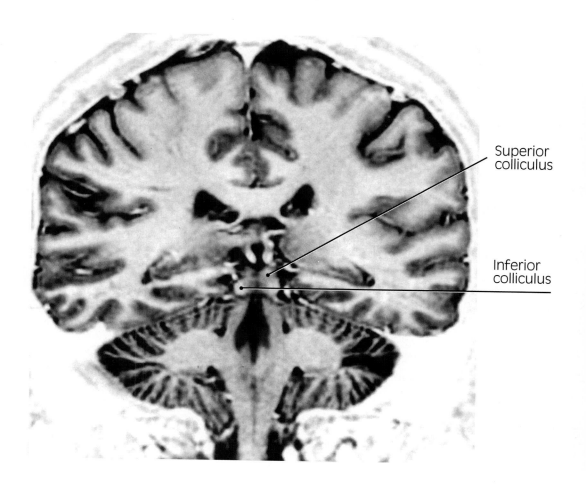

Superior
colliculus

Inferior
colliculus

## Internal Anatomy

We conveniently study the internal structure of the midbrain at the level of the superior and inferior colliculi.

### Internal Anatomy at the Inferior Colliculi

#### Gray Matter

The central periaqueductal gray matter contains:

- The nucleus of the trochlear nerve in the ventromedial part

- A mesencephalic nucleus of the trigeminal nerve in the lateral part

Substantia nigra, a lamina of gray matter, is the largest nucleus of the midbrain found in both the caudal and rostral portions. Nigral cells contain melanin pigments and synthesize dopamine.

#### White Matter

Crus Cerebri

Contents, midline:   Pyramidal tract

Medial one-sixth: Frontopontine fibers

Lateral one-sixth: Temporopontine, parietopontine, and occipitopontine fibers

#### *Tegmentum*

Contents:   Medial, trigeminal, spinal, and lateral lemnisci

Midline decussation of the superior cerebellar peduncles

Medial longitudinal bundle

Tectospinal and rubrospinal tracts

(Figures **7.6** to **7.14**)

Figure **7.6**

Midbrain, axial view, magnified.

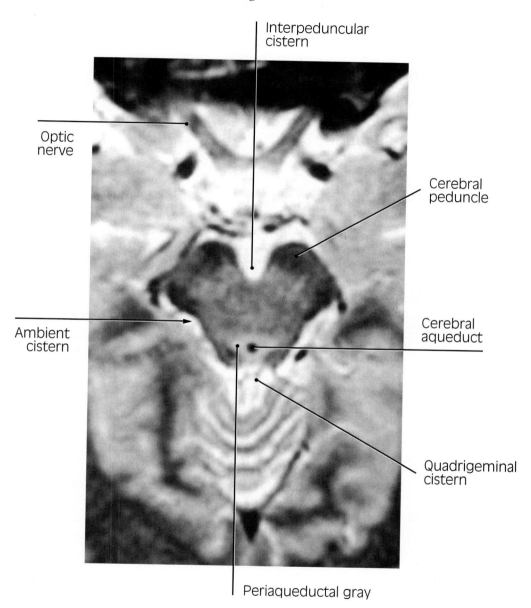

Interpeduncular cistern

Optic nerve

Cerebral peduncle

Ambient cistern

Cerebral aqueduct

Quadrigeminal cistern

Periaqueductal gray

## Internal Anatomy at the Superior Colliculi

### Gray Matter

The central gray matter contains:

- The nucleus of the oculomotor nerve in the ventromedial part
- Mesencephalic nucleus of the trigeminal nerve in the lateral part

Pretectal nucleus

Red nucleus: A large ovoid nucleus in the anterior tegmentum that measures about 5 mm in diameter. It contains iron.

Substantia nigra, with same contents as red nucleus

### White Matter

Crus cerebri and tegmentum, with same contents as red nucleus

Connection of the posterior commissure to the superior colliculi

### PRACTICAL POINTS

Nigral cells of the substantia nigra contain neuromelanine pigment, synthesize dopamine.

The nigrostriatal pathway is highly significant in relation to Parkinson's disease.

The mesolimbic dopaminergic pathway (from the ventral tegmentum to the limbic system) is significant in psychiatric disorders such as schizophrenia.

The red nucleus is the part of the extrapyramidal system.

The central gray matter surrounding the aqueduct is the part of the midbrain reticular formation. The periaqueductal gray matter is bounded on each side by the locus ceruleus, which contains the largest collection of noradrenergic neurons.

The inferior colliculi constitute a relay station of auditory information.

The superior colliculi are primarily a visual reflex center.

A pretectal region is the center for the pupillary light reflex.

Figure **7.7**

Midbrain, axial view, magnified.

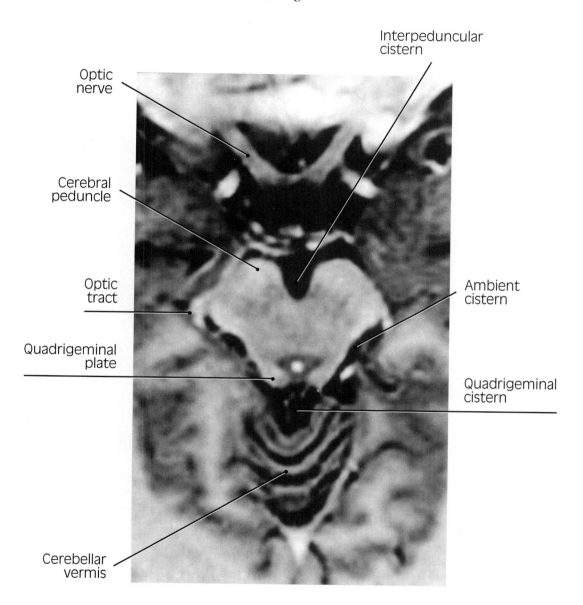

Figure **7.8**

Midbrain, Mickey's anatomy, axial view, magnified.

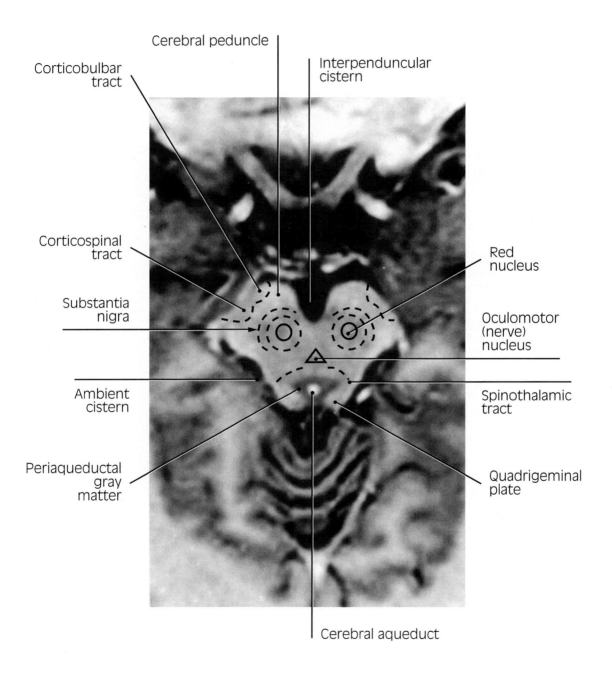

Cerebral peduncle

Corticobulbar tract

Interpenduncular cistern

Corticospinal tract

Red nucleus

Substantia nigra

Oculomotor (nerve) nucleus

Ambient cistern

Spinothalamic tract

Periaqueductal gray matter

Quadrigeminal plate

Cerebral aqueduct

Figure **7.9**

Midbrain, axial view, magnified.

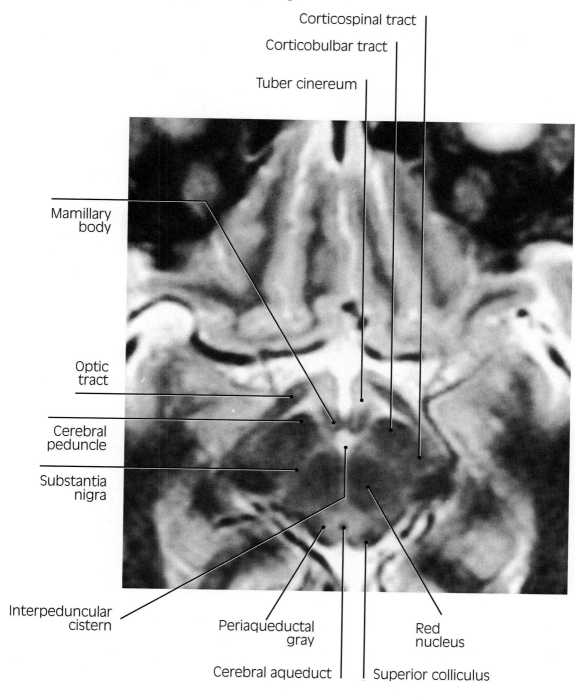

Corticospinal tract

Corticobulbar tract

Tuber cinereum

Mamillary body

Optic tract

Cerebral peduncle

Substantia nigra

Interpeduncular cistern

Periaqueductal gray

Red nucleus

Cerebral aqueduct

Superior colliculus

Figure **7.10**

Midbrain, axial view, magnified.

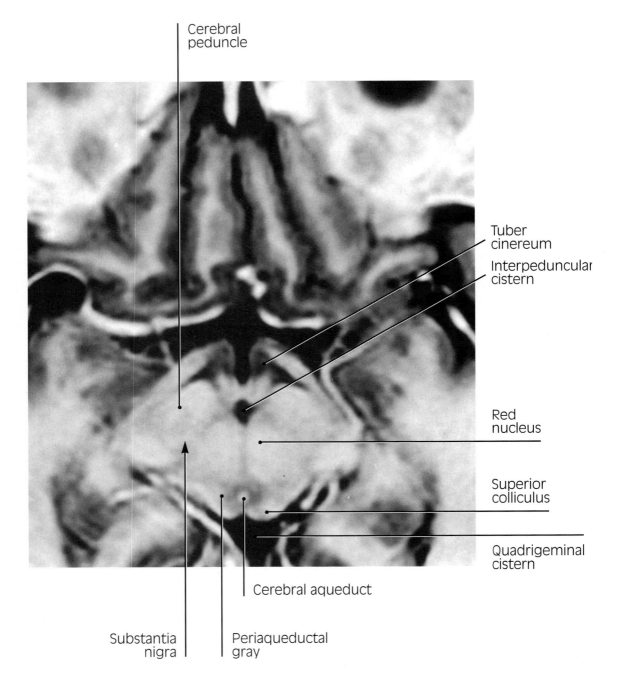

Cerebral peduncle

Tuber cinereum

Interpeduncular cistern

Red nucleus

Superior colliculus

Quadrigeminal cistern

Cerebral aqueduct

Substantia nigra

Periaqueductal gray

Figure **7.11**

Midbrain, axial view, magnified.

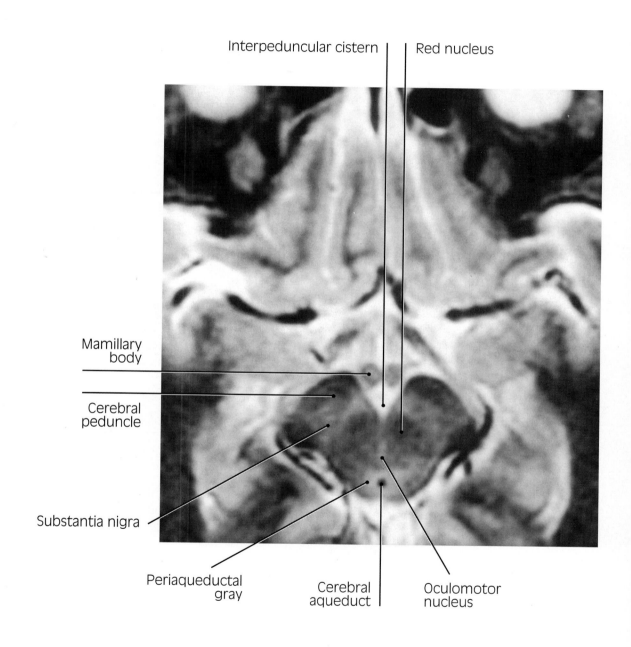

Figure **7.12**

Midbrain, axial view, magnified.

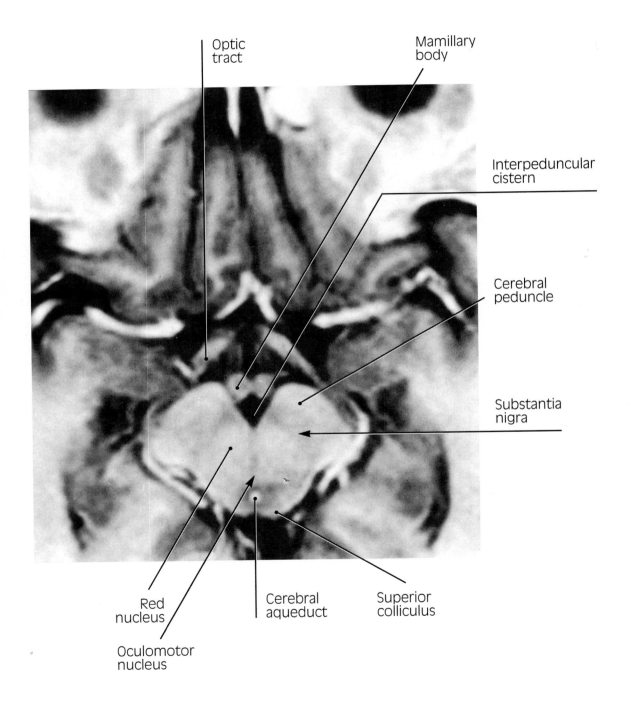

Optic
tract

Mamillary
body

Interpeduncular
cistern

Cerebral
peduncle

Substantia
nigra

Red
nucleus

Oculomotor
nucleus

Cerebral
aqueduct

Superior
colliculus

Figure **7.13**

Midbrain, coronal view.

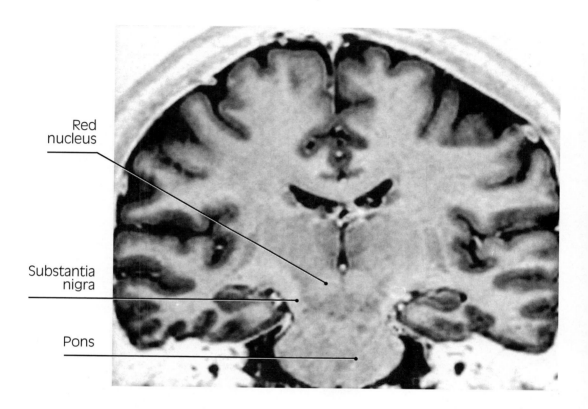

Red
nucleus

Substantia
nigra

Pons

Figure **7.14**

Midbrain, coronal view, magnified.

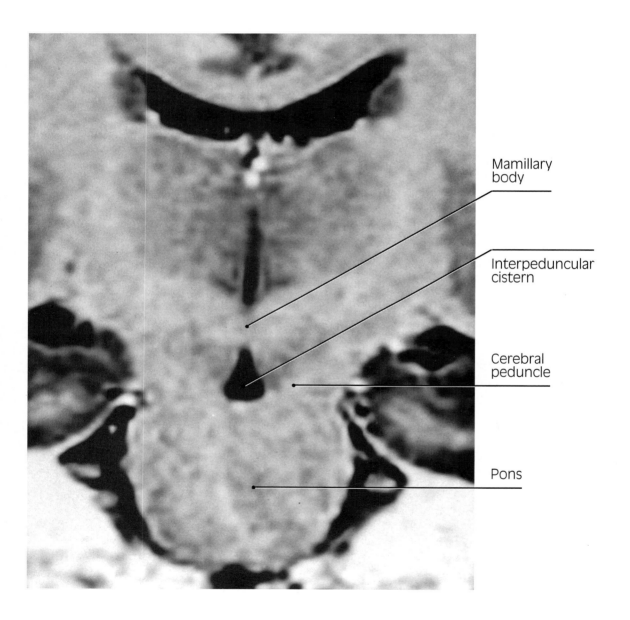

Mamillary body

Interpeduncular cistern

Cerebral peduncle

Pons

CHAPTER **8**

# Metencephalon: Pons

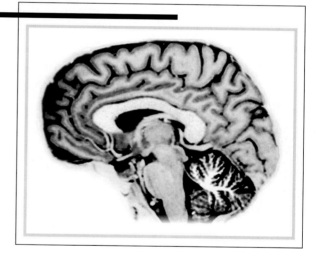

The pons is the middle part of the brain stem, connecting the midbrain with the medulla. The word *pons* means the bridge. The classic "pregnant belly" appearance is shown on the sagittal MR image in (Figure **8.1**).

## Surfaces

Anterior:   Convex in both directions with transverse striations.

The vertical median sulcus lodges the basilar artery.

We see the abducent, facial, and vestibulocochlear nerves attached to the lower border of this surface.

Lateral:   Continuous with the middle cerebral peduncle.

We see the trigeminal nerve attached to this surface at the junction of the pons with the peduncle.

**NOTE** The cerebellum and the upper half of the floors of the fourth ventricle hide the posterior surface of the pons.

## Internal Anatomy

We best study the internal anatomy of the pons in the transverse sections:

- The anterior and basilar parts are continuous inferiorly with the pyramids of the medulla, and on each side with the cerebellum through the middle cerebellar peduncle.

- The dorsal or tegmental part is a direct upward continuation of the medulla, excluding the pyramids.

### Anterior and Basilar Parts

Uniform throughout its length except for the tegmentum of the pons, which is different in the upper and lower parts

Gray matter:   Pontine nuclei

White matter:   Longitudinal pyramidal and transverse pontocerebellar fibers

Figure **8.1**

Pons, sagittal view, magnified.

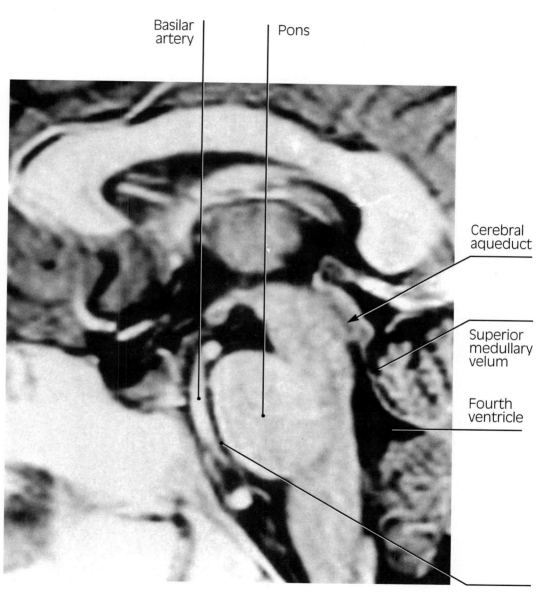

## Tegmentum in the Lower Pons

(Figures **8.2** and **8.3**)

**Gray matter:** Sixth nerve nucleus

Seventh nerve nucleus

Vestibular and cochlear nuclei

Spinal nucleus of the trigeminal nerve

Salivary and lacrimal nuclei

**White matter:** Trapezoid body: Just behind the ventral pons, part of an auditory pathway

Medial lemniscus: Either side of midline, behind the trapezoid body

Lateral spinothalamic tract: Lateral to the medial lemniscus

(Figures **8.4** to **8.6**)

Figure **8.2**

Pons, axial view, magnified.

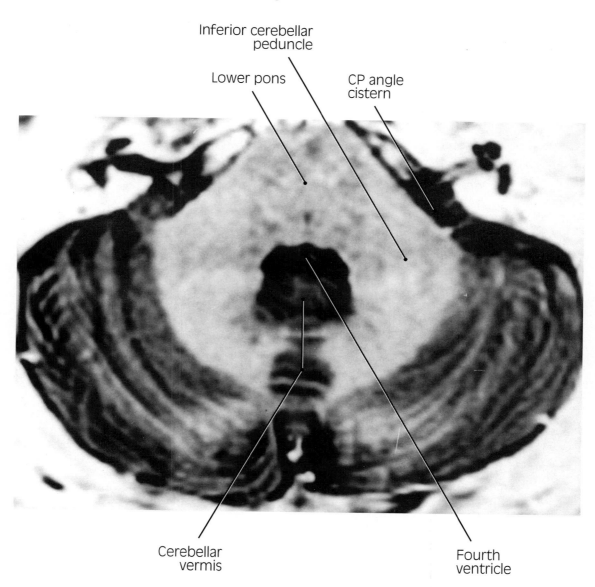

Inferior cerebellar peduncle

Lower pons

CP angle cistern

Cerebellar vermis

Fourth ventricle

Figure **8.3**

Pons, axial view, magnified.

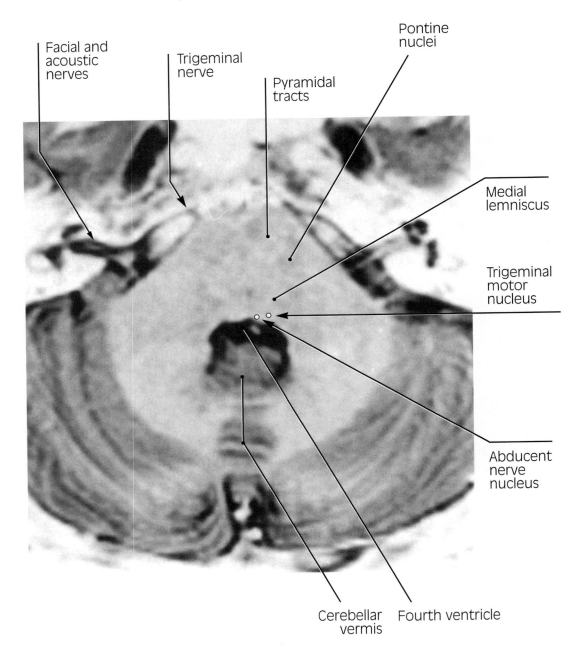

Facial and acoustic nerves

Trigeminal nerve

Pyramidal tracts

Pontine nuclei

Medial lemniscus

Trigeminal motor nucleus

Abducent nerve nucleus

Cerebellar vermis

Fourth ventricle

Figure **8.4**

Pons, axial view, magnified.

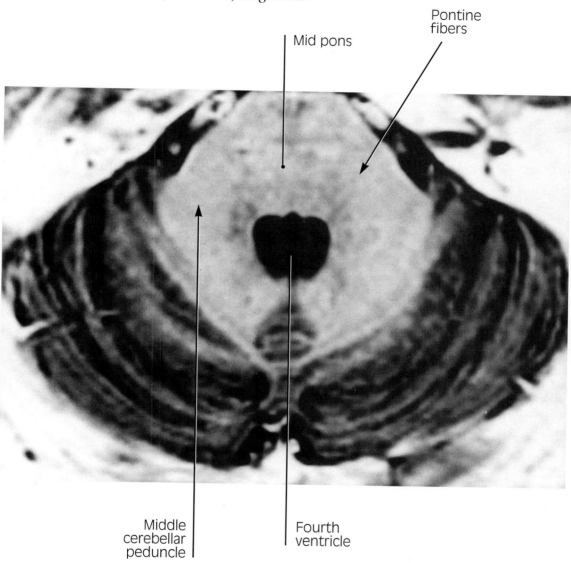

Mid pons

Pontine
fibers

Middle
cerebellar
peduncle

Fourth
ventricle

Figure **8.5**

Pons, axial view, magnified.

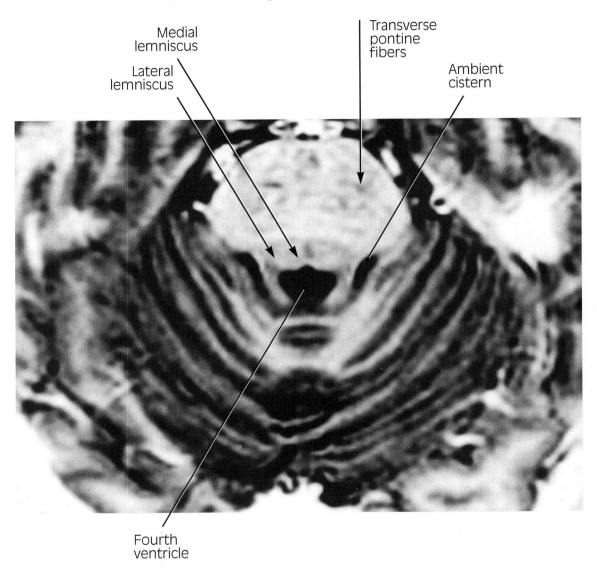

Medial
lemniscus

Lateral
lemniscus

Transverse
pontine
fibers

Ambient
cistern

Fourth
ventricle

Figure **8.6**

## Pons, axial view, magnified.

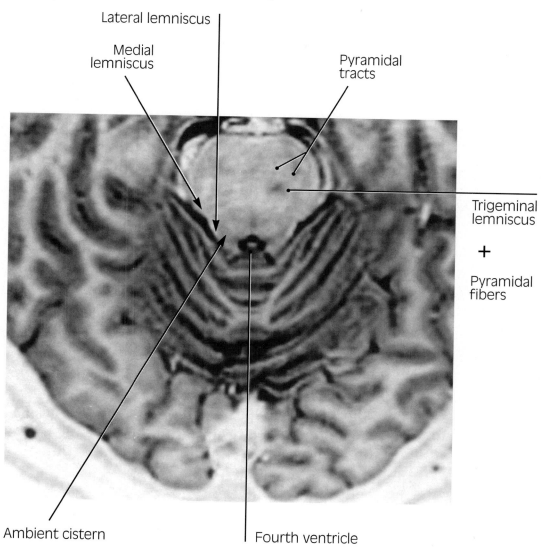

Lateral lemniscus

Medial lemniscus

Pyramidal tracts

Trigeminal lemniscus

**+**

Pyramidal fibers

Ambient cistern

Fourth ventricle

## Tegmentum in the Upper Pons

(Figures **8.7** to **8.9**)

Gray matter:    Motor and superior sensory nuclei of the trigeminal nerve

White matter:    Lateral sides of the medial lemniscus

Trigeminal lemniscus

Lateral lemniscus

The medial longitudinal bundle interconnects the nuclei of the oculomotor, trochlear, trigeminal, abducent, and the spinal part of the accessory nerves.

### PRACTICAL POINT

A unilateral lesion in the lower pons results in facial paralysis on the side of the lesion and hemiplegia on the opposite side (crossed hemiplegia or Millard-Gubler syndrome).

Figure **8.7**

Pons, axial view, magnified.

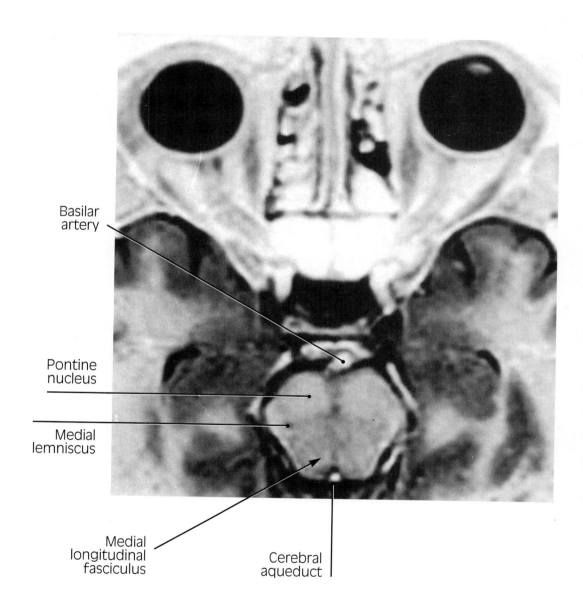

Basilar
artery

Pontine
nucleus

Medial
lemniscus

Medial
longitudinal
fasciculus

Cerebral
aqueduct

Figure **8.8**

Pons, axial view, magnified.

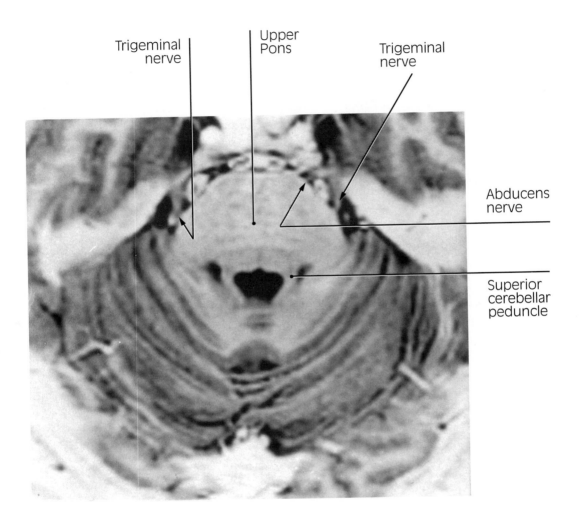

Trigeminal nerve

Upper Pons

Trigeminal nerve

Abducens nerve

Superior cerebellar peduncle

Figure **8.9**

Pons, coronal view.

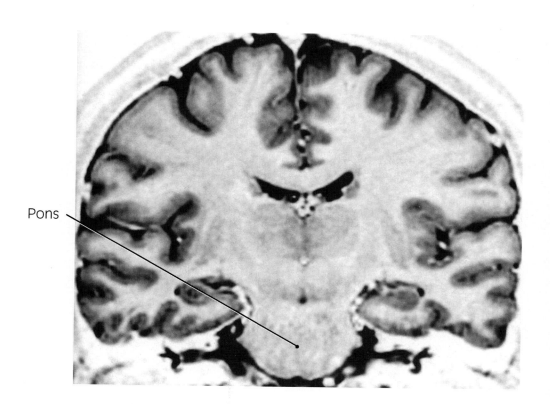

Pons

# CHAPTER 9

# Metencephalon: Cerebellum

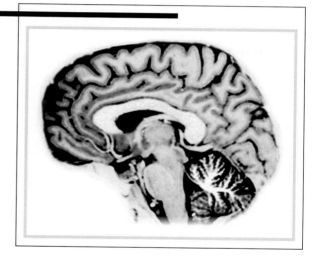

(Figure **9.1**)

## Location

In the posterior cranial fossa, behind the pons and medulla

## Relationships

Anterior:   Fourth ventricle

             Pons

             Medulla

Posterior:   Squamous occipital bone

Inferior:   Squamous occipital bone

Superior:   Tentorium cerebelli or the dural folds

## Anatomy

Complex

## Main Segments

Vermis

Hemispheres

## Surfaces

Superior:   Convex

Inferior:   Deep median notch, or the vallecula

Superior and lateral:   Flocculus (seen as a bump, a potential pseudotumor) extends to the cerebellopontine angle cistern

Inferior and lateral:   Tonsils (important for Chiari malformations) (Figures **9.2** and **9.3**)

The two cerebellar hemispheres are united to each other through a median vermis, while separated by the vallecula.

Figure **9.1**

Cerebellum, sagittal view, magnified.

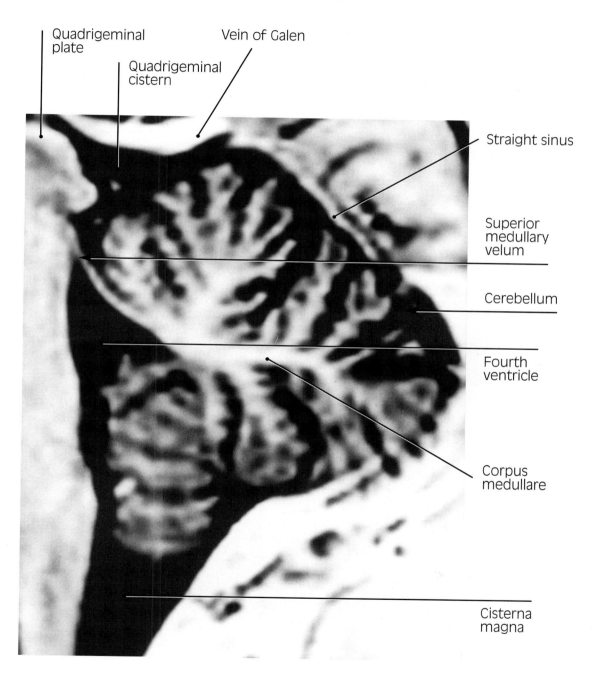

Quadrigeminal plate

Quadrigeminal cistern

Vein of Galen

Straight sinus

Superior medullary velum

Cerebellum

Fourth ventricle

Corpus medullare

Cisterna magna

Figure **9.2**

Cerebellum (tonsils) and medulla, axial view, magnified.

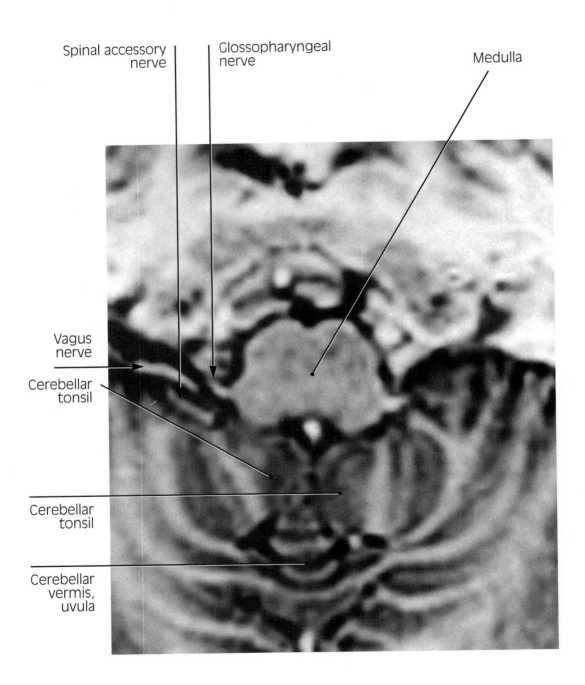

Spinal accessory nerve

Glossopharyngeal nerve

Medulla

Vagus nerve

Cerebellar tonsil

Cerebellar tonsil

Cerebellar vermis, uvula

Figure **9.3**

Cerebellar tonsils, coronal view, magnified.

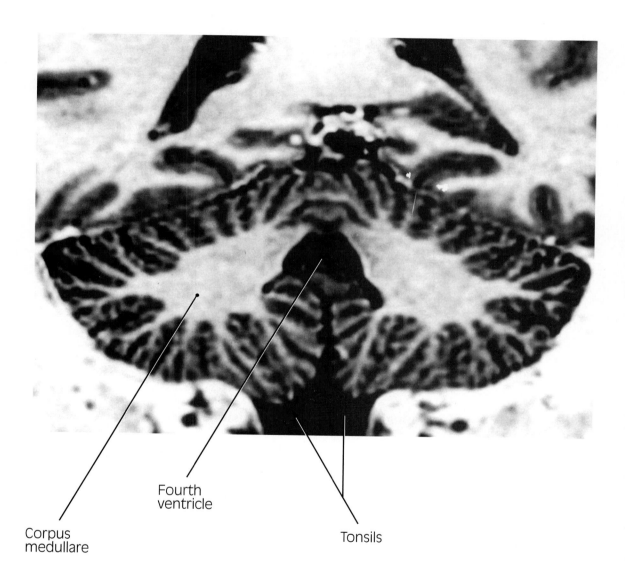

Corpus
medullare

Fourth
ventricle

Tonsils

## Vermis, Divisions
(Figures **9.4** to **9.10**)

| Superior Surface | Inferior Surface |
|---|---|
| Lingula | Tuber |
| Central | Pyramid |
| Culmen | Uvula |
| Declive | Nodule |
| Folium | |

## Cerebellar Hemispheres

### Anatomic Divisions

| Lobes | Location | Generation | Size | Dividing Fissure |
|---|---|---|---|---|
| Anterior | Superior | More recent | Medium | Fissura prima |
| Middle | Posterior | Most recent | Largest | Fissura prima superiorly and posterolateral fissure inferiorly |
| Flocculonodular | Inferior | Oldest | Smallest | |

### Morphologic and Functional Divisions

| Morphology | Generation | Lobes | Connections | Functions |
|---|---|---|---|---|
| Archicerebellum | Oldest | Flocculonodular and lingula | Vestibular | Equilibrium |
| Paleocerebellum | More recent | Anterior (no lingula) Uvula Pyramid | Spino-cerebellar | Tone, posture, and crude movements |
| Neocerebellum | Most recent | Middle (no uvula and pyramid) | Cortico-cerebellar | Fine movements |

Figure **9.4**

Cerebellum, vermis, fissures, sagittal view, magnified.

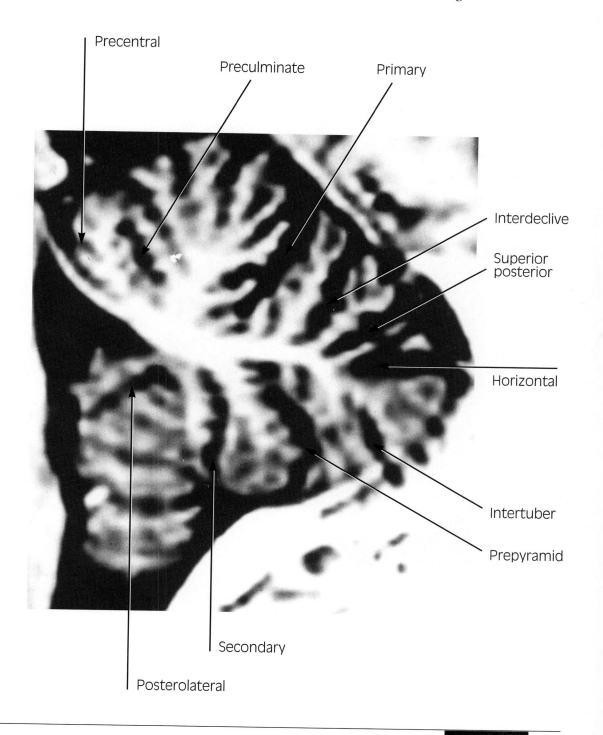

Figure **9.5**

Cerebellum, vermis (segments), sagittal view, magnified.

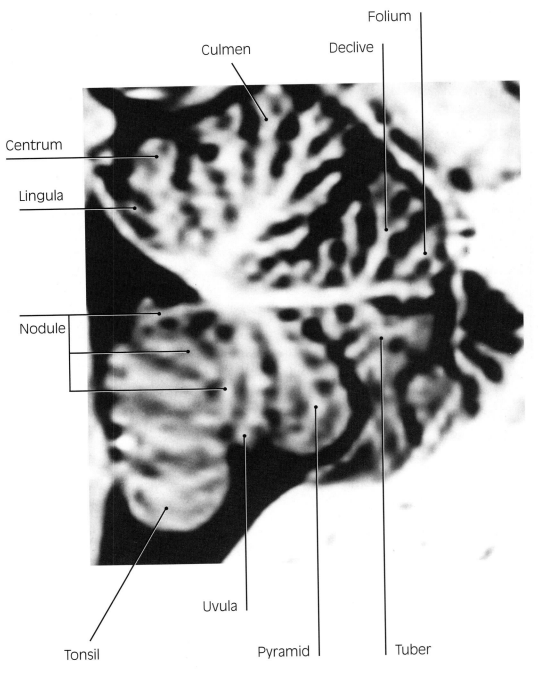

Figure **9.6**

Cerebellum, vermis, axial view, magnified.

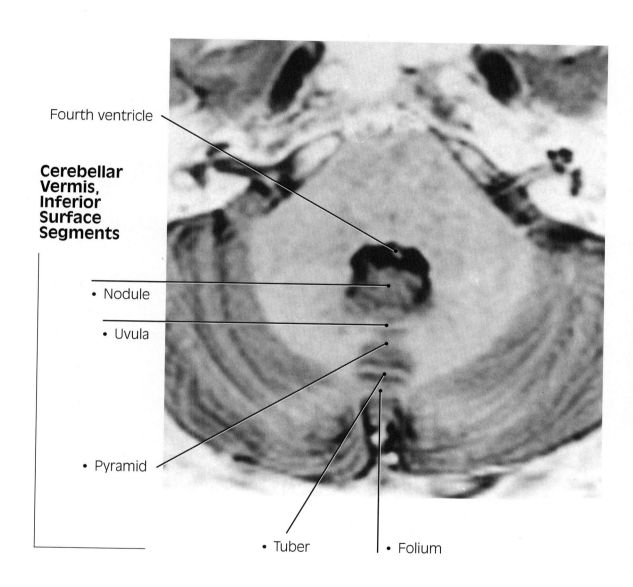

Fourth ventricle

**Cerebellar
Vermis,
Inferior
Surface
Segments**

- Nodule

- Uvula

- Pyramid

- Tuber

- Folium

Figure **9.7**

Cerebellum, axial view, magnified.

Pons

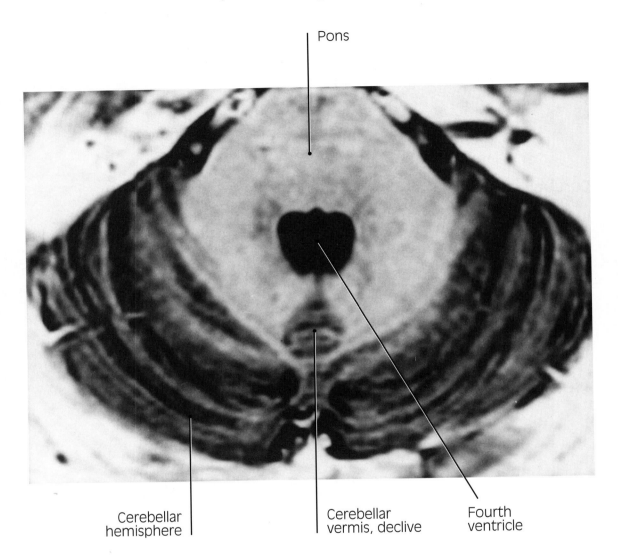

Cerebellar
hemisphere

Cerebellar
vermis, declive

Fourth
ventricle

Figure **9.8**

Cerebellum, vermis, axial view, magnified.

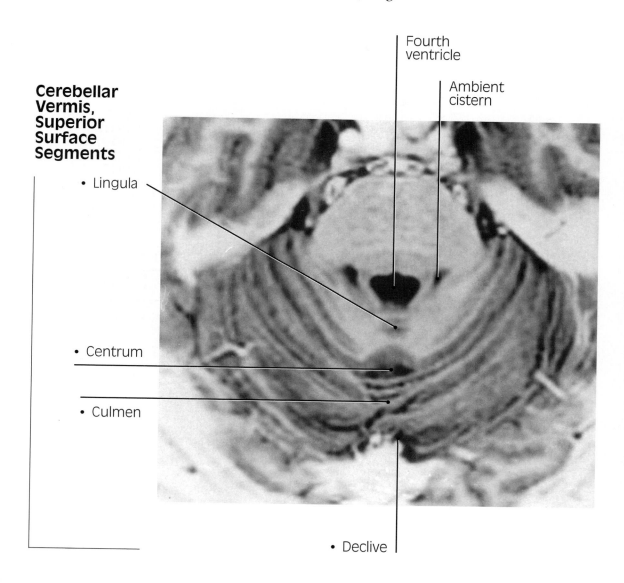

Fourth
ventricle

Ambient
cistern

**Cerebellar
Vermis,
Superior
Surface
Segments**

• Lingula

• Centrum

• Culmen

• Declive

Figure **9.9**

Cerebellum, vermis, axial view, magnified.

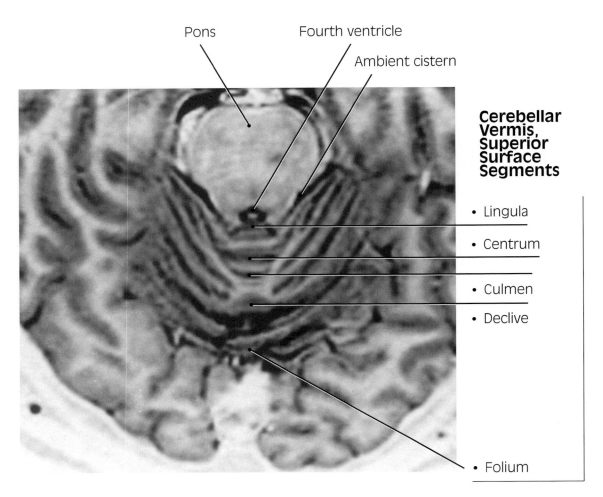

Pons    Fourth ventricle

Ambient cistern

**Cerebellar Vermis, Superior Surface Segments**

- Lingula
- Centrum
- Culmen
- Declive
- Folium

Figure **9.10**

Cerebellar hemisphere, coronal view, magnified.

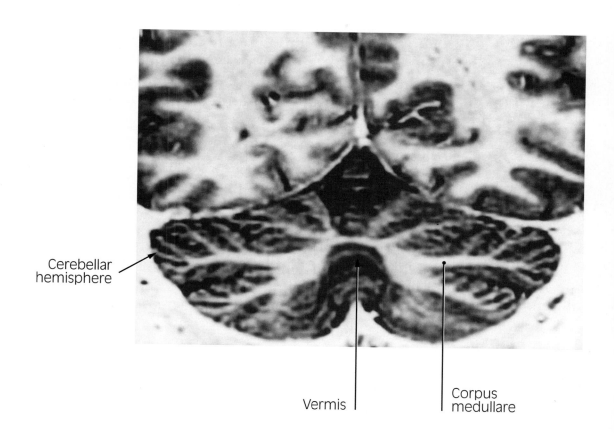

Cerebellar
hemisphere

Vermis

Corpus
medullare

## Morphologic Divisions and Nuclei

| Morphologic Divisions | Nuclei | Matter |
|---|---|---|
| Archicerebellar | Fastigii | Gray |
| Paleocerebellar | Globosus | Gray |
| | Emboliformis | Gray |
| Neocerebellar | Dentate | White |

## Further Subdivisions

(Figures **9.11** to **9.15**)

Lobules superior to inferior with separating fissures as follows:

Ala

Quadrangular lobule

Primary fissure

Simple lobule

Superior semilunar lobule

Horizontal fissure

Inferior semilunar lobule

Gracile lobule

Biventral lobule

Tonsil

Posterolateral fissure

Flocculus

Figure **9.11**

Cerebellar hemisphere, sagittal view, magnified.

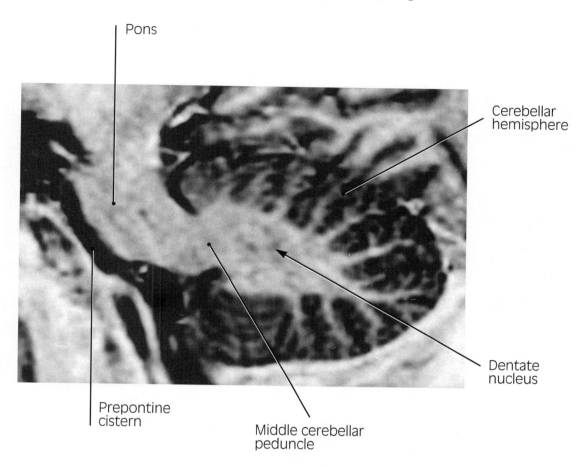

Pons

Cerebellar
hemisphere

Dentate
nucleus

Prepontine
cistern

Middle cerebellar
peduncle

Figure **9.12**

Cerebellum, sagittal view, magnified.

Midbrain

Pons

Middle
cerebellar
peduncle

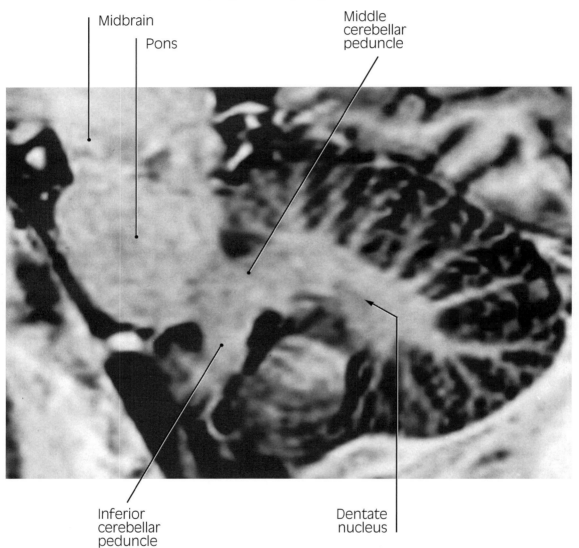

Inferior
cerebellar
peduncle

Dentate
nucleus

Figure **9.13**

Cerebellar hemisphere, lobes, sagittal view, magnified.

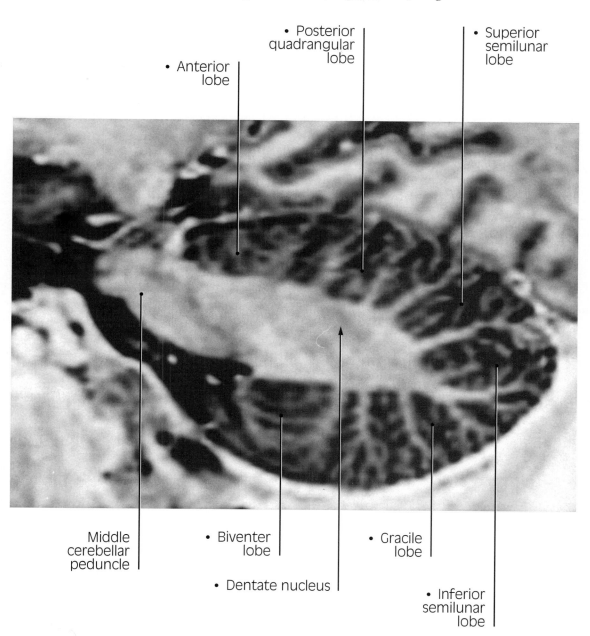

- Anterior lobe
- Posterior quadrangular lobe
- Superior semilunar lobe
- Middle cerebellar peduncle
- Biventer lobe
- Gracile lobe
- Dentate nucleus
- Inferior semilunar lobe

Figure **9.14**

Cerebellar hemisphere, fissures, sagittal view, magnified.

Primary
fissure

Superior
posterior
fissure

Horizontal
fissure

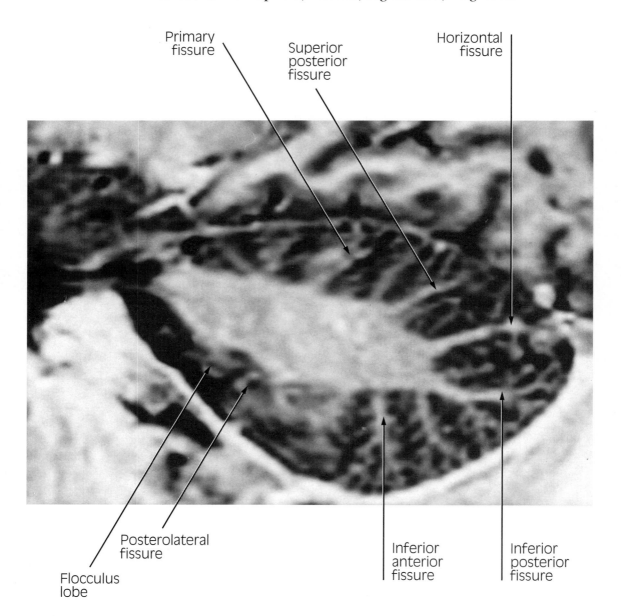

Posterolateral
fissure

Flocculus
lobe

Inferior
anterior
fissure

Inferior
posterior
fissure

Figure **9.15**

Cerebellar hemisphere, lobes, coronal view, magnified.

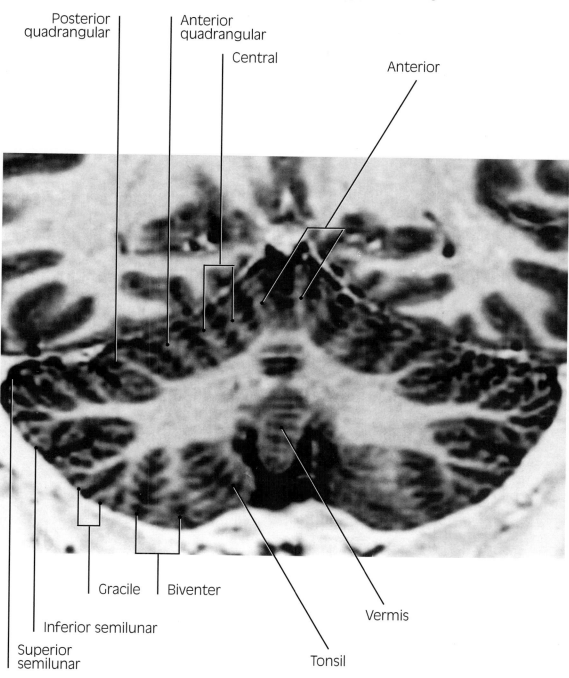

Posterior quadrangular

Anterior quadrangular

Central

Anterior

Gracile

Biventer

Vermis

Inferior semilunar

Superior semilunar

Tonsil

## Cerebellar White Matter Tracts: Cerebellar Peduncles

(Figures **9.16** and **9.17**)

| Cerebellar Peduncles | Synonym | Connection |
| --- | --- | --- |
| Superior | Brachium conjunctivum | Midbrain to cerebellum |
| Middle | Brachium pontis | Pons to cerebellum |
| Inferior | Restiform body | Medulla to cerebellum |

Figure **9.16**

Cerebellar peduncles, coronal view, magnified.

Superior
cerebellar peduncle

Corpus
medullare

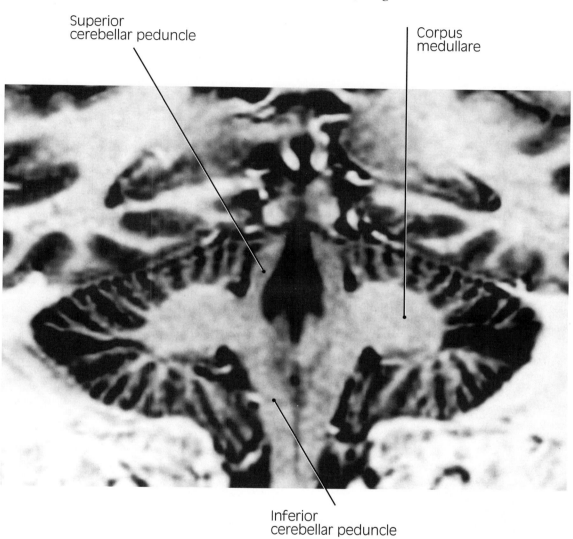

Inferior
cerebellar peduncle

Figure **9.17**

Cerebellar peduncles, coronal view, magnified.

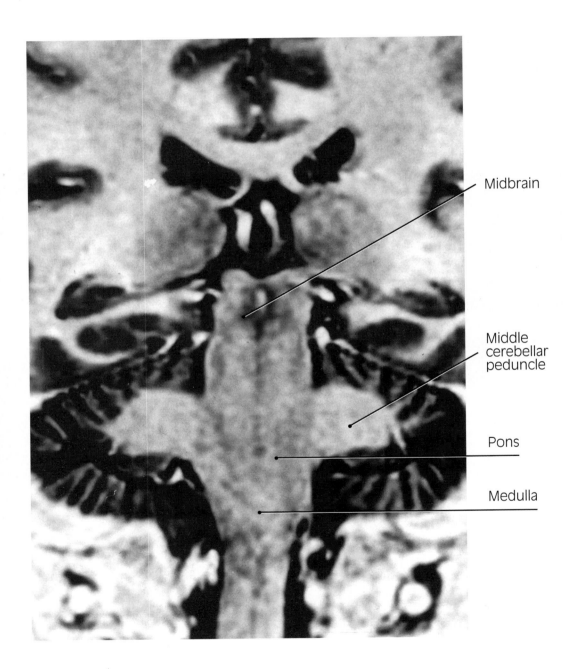

Midbrain

Middle cerebellar peduncle

Pons

Medulla

# CHAPTER 10

# Myelencephalon:
# Medulla

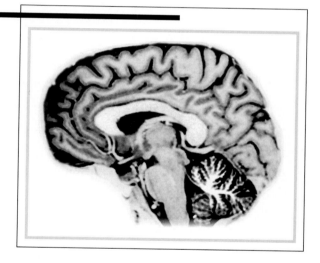

The medulla is the lowest part of the brain stem. It extends from the lower border of the pons to a plane just above the first cervical nerve, where it is continuous with the spinal cord.

## External Anatomy

(Figures **10.1** to **10.3**)

### Divisions

Right and left by the anterior and posterior median fissures

Each half further divided into anterior, lateral, and posterior regions by the anterolateral and posterolateral sulci

**Anterior region:**    The pyramid: Longitudinal elevation

Contents: Corticospinal fibers

Pyramidal decussation: In the lower medulla

**Anterolateral sulcus:**    Rootlets of hypoglossal nerve between the pyramid and olive

**Lateral region:**    Olive: Upper lateral oval elevation

Contents: Gray mass of inferior olivary nucleus

**Posterolateral sulcus:**    Rootlets of glossopharyngeal, vagus, and cranial part of accessory nerves

Figure **10.1**

Medulla, sagittal view, magnified.

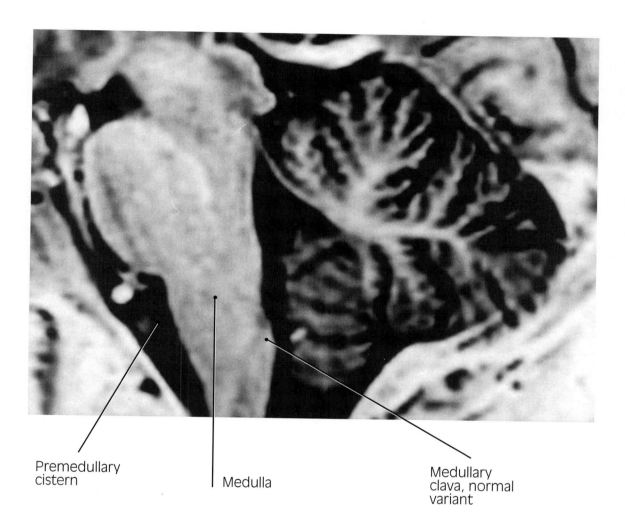

Premedullary
cistern

Medulla

Medullary
clava, normal
variant

**Posterolateral region:**   Upper part: V-shaped depression, corresponds to the floor of the fourth ventricle

Below the floor of the fourth ventricle are three longitudinal elevations from medial to lateral sides, as follow:

- Fasciculus gracilis, houses the nucleus gracilis

- Fasciculus cuneatus, houses the nucleus cuneatus

- Inferior cerebellar peduncle

**N O T E**   The nucleus gracilis and cuneatus are seen as tubercles at the upper end.

**Lower medulla:**   Tuber Cinerium: Elevation lateral to the Fasciculus Cuneatus

Houses mass of gray matter of spinal nucleus of the trigeminal nerve

Figure **10.2**

Medulla, coronal view, magnified.

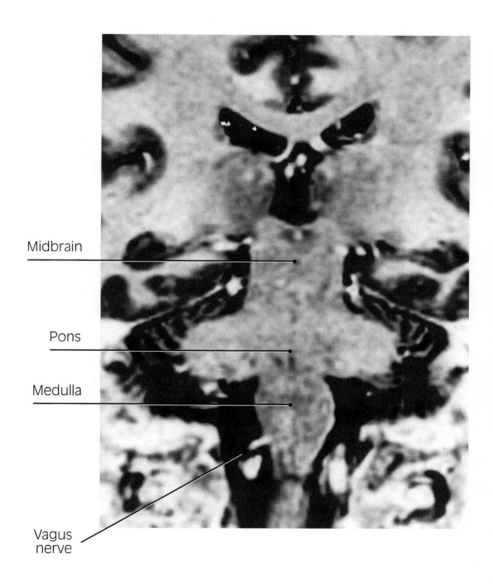

Midbrain

Pons

Medulla

Vagus
nerve

# Internal Anatomy

We best study the internal anatomy in the transverse sections.

## Internal Anatomy at the Lower, Mid, and Upper Medullary Regions

|  | Lower Medulla | Mid Medulla | Upper Medulla |
|---|---|---|---|
| Decussation | Pyramidal | Sensory | — |
| Gray matter<br>• Nuclei | Central gray with<br>• Gracilis<br>• Cuneatus | Central gray with<br>• Hypoglossal<br>• Dorsal vagal<br>• Tractus solitarius | Central gray with<br>• Hypoglossal<br>• Dorsal vagal<br>• Tractus Solitarius<br>• Inferior and medial vestibular |
|  |  | Accessory cuneate | Medial and dorsal accessory olivary |
|  | Lateral gray with spinal tract of trigeminal nerve | Spinal tract of trigeminal nerve | Spinal tract of trigeminal nerve |
|  |  | Lower part of inferior olivary | Inferior olivary |
|  |  |  | Ambiguus |
|  |  |  | Dorsal and ventral cochlear |
|  |  |  | Arcuate |
| White matter | Pyramids + decussation | Medial lemniscus | Inferior cerebellar peduncle |
|  | Fasciculus gracilis | Pyramidal tract | Olivocerebellar tract |
|  | Fasciculus cuneatus | Medial longitudinal bundle | Striae medullares |
|  |  | Spinocerebellar and lateral spinothalamic tracts |  |

Figure **10.3**

Medulla, axial view.

**Cranial Nerves**

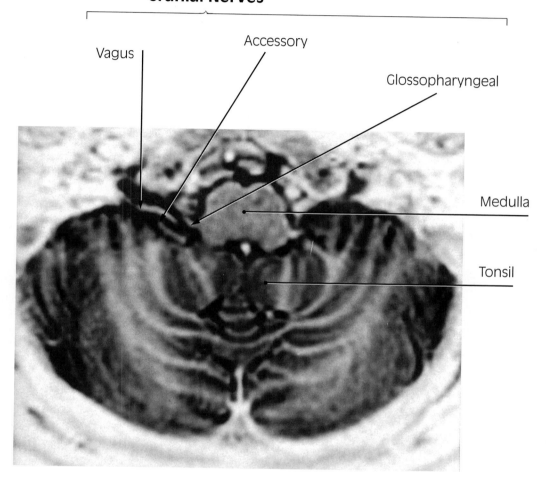

## Nuclear Arrangements in the Upper Medulla in the Floor of the Fourth Ventricle

(Figure **10.4**)

**Hypoglossal:**   Paramedian position

**Dorsal vagal:**   Lateral to hypoglossal

**Tractus solitarius:**   Ventrolateral to dorsal vagal

**Inferior and medial vestibular:**   Medial to inferior cerebellar peduncle

**Ambiguus:**   Deep in the reticular formation of the medulla

**Dorsal and ventral cochlear:**   On the surface of the inferior cerebellar peduncle

**Spinal tract of the trigeminal nerve:**   Dorsolateral part

**Arcuate:**   Anteromedial to the pyramidal tract

### FUNCTIONAL CONSIDERATIONS

Injury to the medulla is usually fatal because of the vital respiratory and vasomotor centers.

Bulbar paralysis of the muscles supplied by the last four cranial nerves.

Medullary syndromes are due to vascular lesions of the vertebral and posterior inferior cerebellar arteries.

Figure **10.4**

Medulla, axial view, magnified.

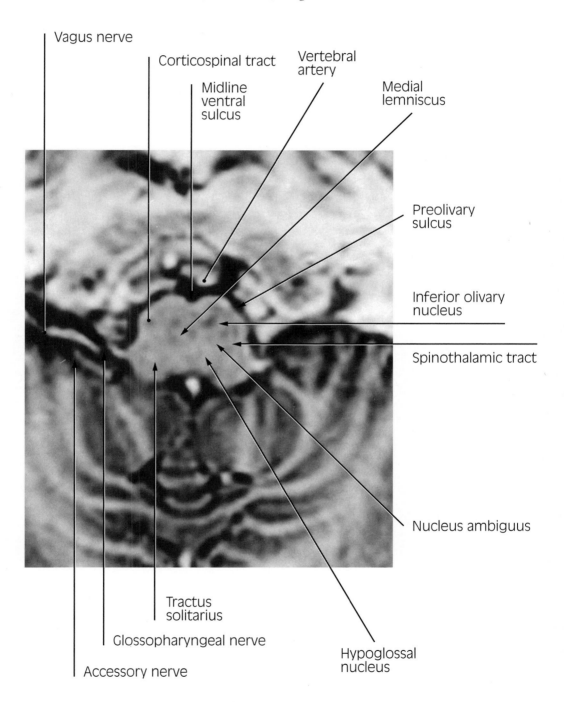

# CHAPTER 11

# Cerebral
# White Matter

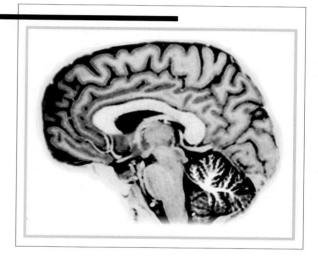

The cerebral white matter consists mainly of the myelinated fibers that connect different parts of the cortex to the other parts of the central nervous system.

# Classification of White Matter Fibers

Association

Projection

Commissural

## Association Fibers

| Type | Subdivisions | Connections |
|------|-------------|-------------|
| Short | — | Adjacent gyri to one another |
| Long | Uncinate fasciculus | Temporal pole to: Motor speech area |
| | | Orbital cortex |
| | Cingulum | Cingulate gyrus to: Parahippocampal gyrus |
| | Superior longitudinal fasciculus | Frontal lobes to: Occipital and temporal lobes |
| | Inferior longitudinal fasciculus | Occipital lobe to: Temporal lobe |

## Projection Fibers

| Type | Connections |
|------|-------------|
| Corticopontine tract | Brain stem to: Spinal cord |
| Corticospinal tract | Brain stem to: Spinal cord |

## Commissural Fibers

(Figure 11.1)

Figure **11.1**

White matter tracts, corpus callosum, anterior and posterior commissures, sagittal view, magnified.

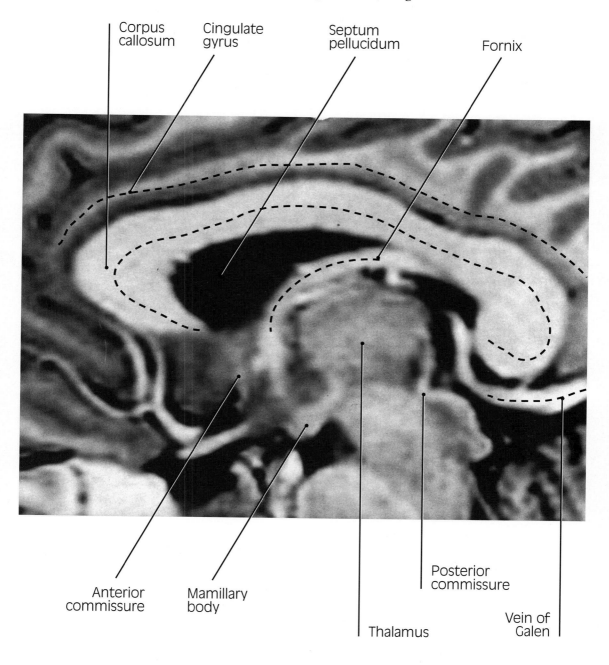

Corpus callosum

Cingulate gyrus

Septum pellucidum

Fornix

Anterior commissure

Mamillary body

Posterior commissure

Thalamus

Vein of Galen

| Type | Connections |
|---|---|
| Corpus callosum | Cerebral cortex of each side |
| Rostrum | Orbital surfaces of the frontal lobes |
| Genu | Two frontal lobes |
| Splenium | Two occipital lobes |
| Anterior commissure | Olfactory bulbs, piriform cortex, and anterior portion of the temporal lobe of either side |
| Posterior commissure | Superior colliculi of each side |
| | Pretectal nucleus of one side to the Edinger-Westphal nucleus of the opposite side |
| Hippocampal or forniceal commissure | Hippocampal formation of each side |
| Habenular commissure | Habenular nuclei of either side |
| Hypothalamic commissure | Anterior hypothalamic commissure of Ganser |
| | Ventral supraoptic commissure of Gudden |
| | Dorsal supraoptic commissure of Meynert |

## Corpus Callosum

(Figures **11.2** to **11.10**)

The largest commissure of the brain that connects the two cerebral hemispheres.

**Length:** Approximately 10 cm

**Location:** Medial surface of the brain in the midline

**Parts:** Genu

Rostrum

Body

Splenium

### Genu

The anterior end is 4 cm behind the frontal pole.

Fibers from the genu form the forceps minor that connects the frontal lobes.

**Relationships:** Anterior: Anterior cerebral arteries

Posterior: Anterior horn of the lateral ventricle

Figure **11.2**

White matter tracts, corpus callosum, parts,
sagittal view, magnified.

- Genu
- Body

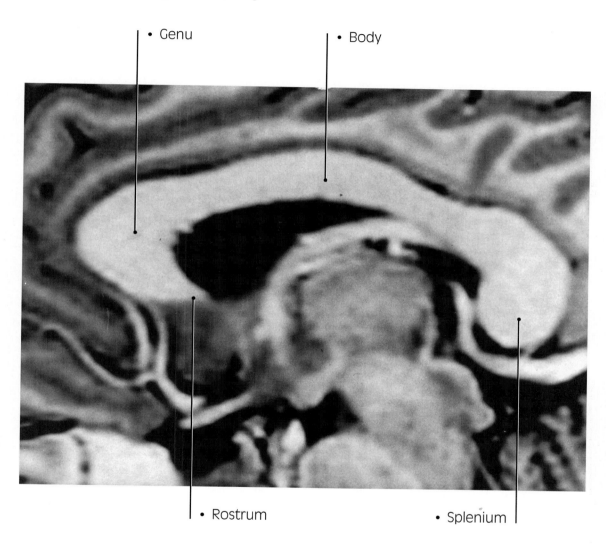

- Rostrum
- Splenium

Figure **11.3**

White matter tracts, corpus callosum, parts,
sagittal view, magnified.

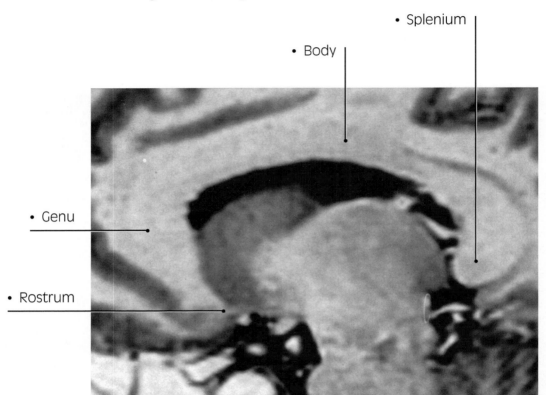

• Splenium

• Body

• Genu

• Rostrum

Figure **11.4**

White matter tracts, corpus callosum, parts, axial view, magnified.

- Corpus callosum, genu

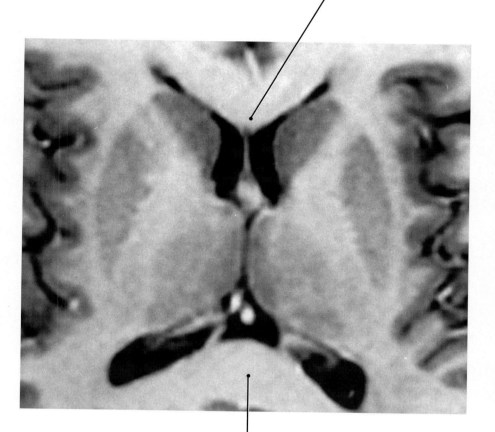

- Corpus callosum, splenium

Figure **11.5**

White matter tracts, corpus callosum, parts, axial view, magnified.

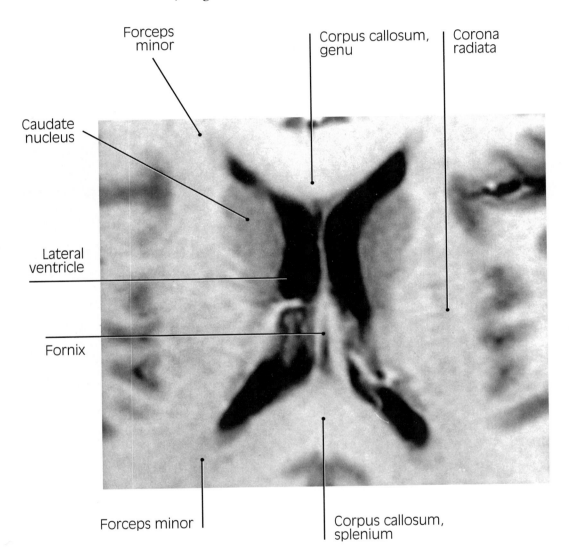

Forceps minor

Corpus callosum, genu

Corona radiata

Caudate nucleus

Lateral ventricle

Fornix

Forceps minor

Corpus callosum, splenium

Figure **11.6**

White matter tracts, corpus callosum, axial view.

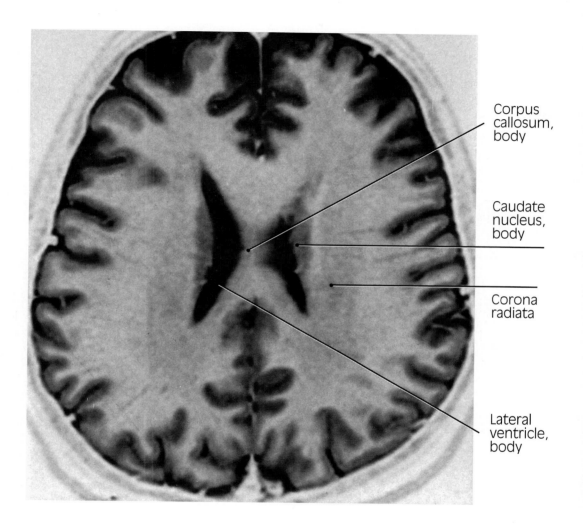

Corpus callosum, body

Caudate nucleus, body

Corona radiata

Lateral ventricle, body

Figure **11.7**

White matter tracts, corpus callosum, axial view.

Corpus
callosum,
body

Lateral
ventricle,
body

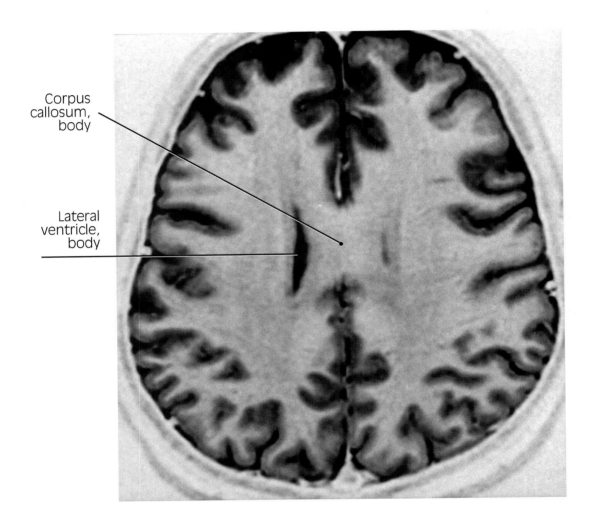

Figure **11.8**

White matter tracts, corpus callosum, coronal view.

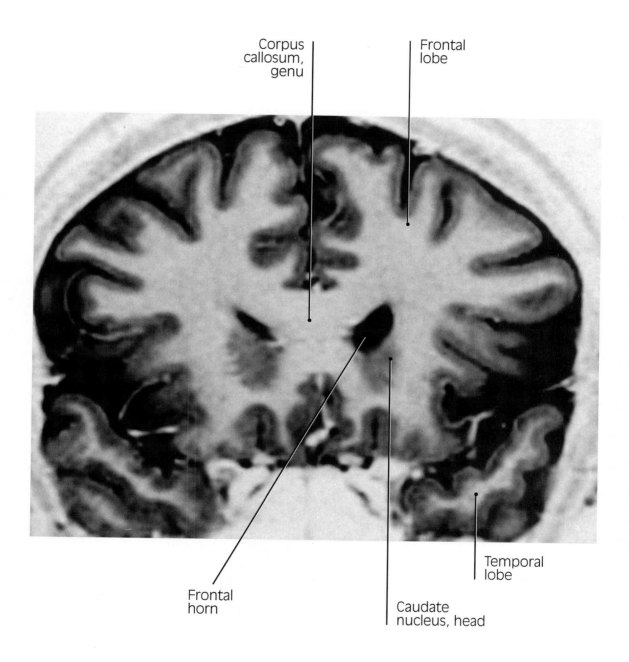

Figure **11.9**

White matter tracts, corpus callosum, body,
coronal view, magnified.

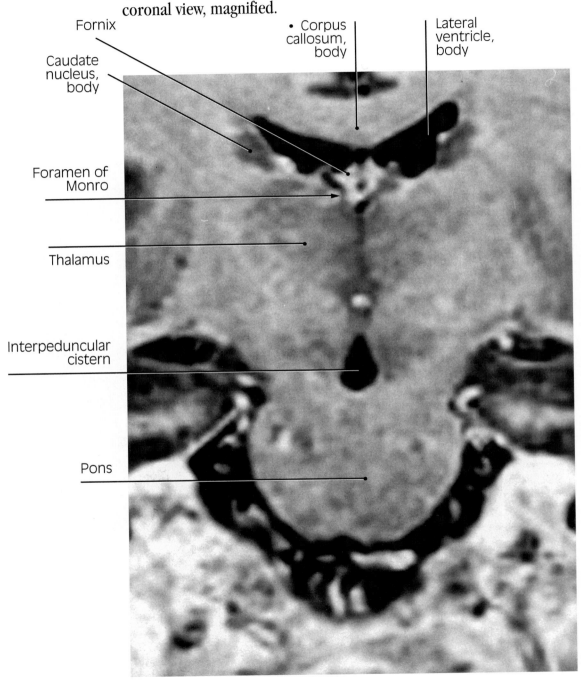

Fornix

Caudate
nucleus,
body

• Corpus
callosum,
body

Lateral
ventricle,
body

Foramen of
Monro

Thalamus

Interpeduncular
cistern

Pons

Figure **11.10**

White matter tracts, corpus callosum, splenium, coronal view, magnified.

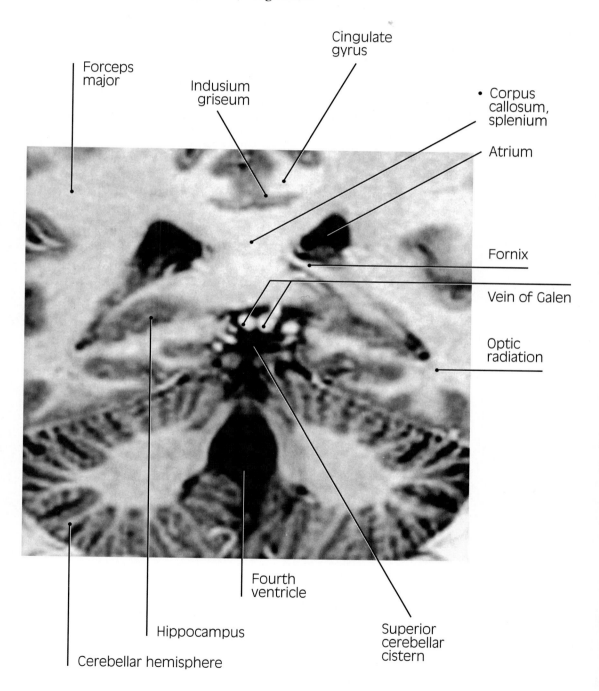

### Rostrum

Directed downward and backward from the genu, and ends by joining the lamina terminalis in front of the anterior commissure, which connects the orbital surfaces of the frontal lobes.

Relationships:    Superior: Anterior horn of the lateral ventricle

Inferior: Longitudinal stria

### Body

Middle portion between the genu and the splenium, overlapped by the gyrus cingulate and covered by the indusium and the longitudinal stria. It forms the roof of the central part of the lateral ventricle.

Superior surface:    Convex from before backward and concave sideways

Inferior surface:    Concave from before backward and convex sideways

Fibers from the body and splenium form the tapetum.

### Splenium

The posterior end, the thickest part of the corpus callosum. It is approximately 6 cm from the occipital pole.

Fibers from the splenium form the forceps major, which connects the occipital lobes.

Relationships:    Superior: Inferior sagittal sinus

Falx cerebri

Inferior: Tela choroidea

Pulvinar

Pineal body

Tectum

Posterior: Great cerebral vein

Straight sinus

Tentorium cerebelli

### Other Commissures

The anterior commissure is between the lamina terminalis and the column of the fornix (Figures **11.11** and **11.12**).

The posterior commissure is just anterior to the pineal gland near the habenula.

The hippocampal or forniceal commissure is between the fornices and ventral to the splenium of the corpus callosum.

Figure **11.11**

White matter tracts, anterior and posterior
commissures, sagittal view, magnified.

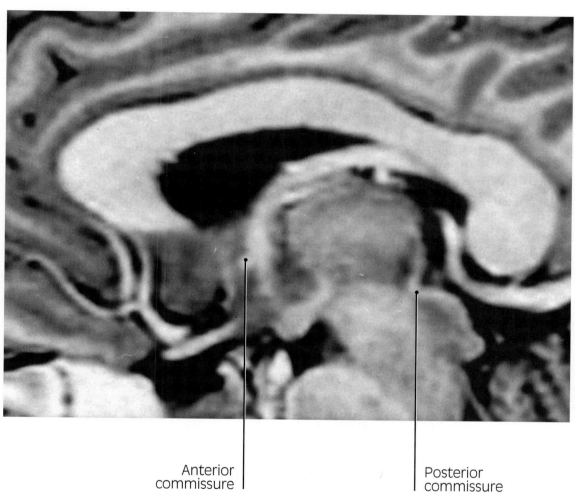

Anterior
commissure

Posterior
commissure

Figure **11.12**

White matter tracts, coronal view.

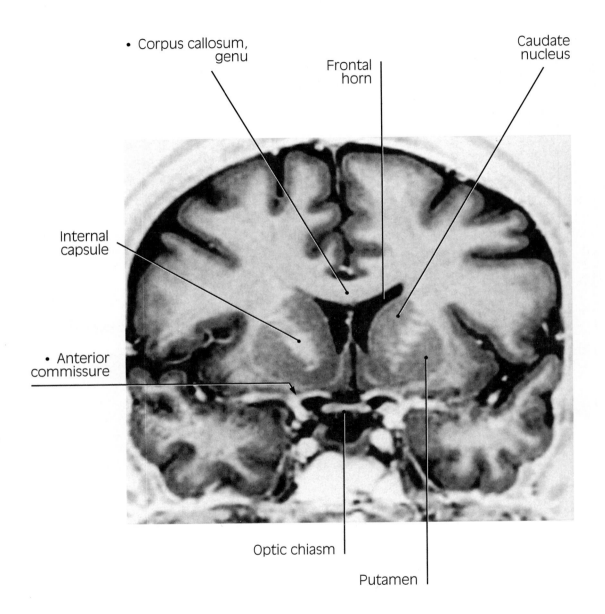

Corpus callosum, genu

Frontal horn

Caudate nucleus

Internal capsule

Anterior commissure

Optic chiasm

Putamen

# CHAPTER 12

# Internal Capsule

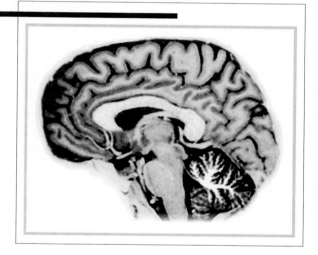

The internal capsule is the principal communication link between the cerebral cortex, the brain stem, and the spinal cord. This vital area consists of a large band of the white matter fibers found between the thalamus, the caudate nucleus, and the putamen. The fibers of the capsule diverge upward and are continuous with the corona radiata, while downward these fibers are continuous with the crus cerebri of the midbrain.

(Figures **12.1** to **12.3**)

**Shape:**    V-shaped, with its concavity directed laterally

## FUNCTIONAL CONSIDERATION

The internal capsule is a narrow path consisting of the densely packed fibers of various important pathways. Therefore, small lesions of the capsule can produce widespread derangements of the body.

29

.1

Capsules, internal, external, and extreme,
axial view, magnified.

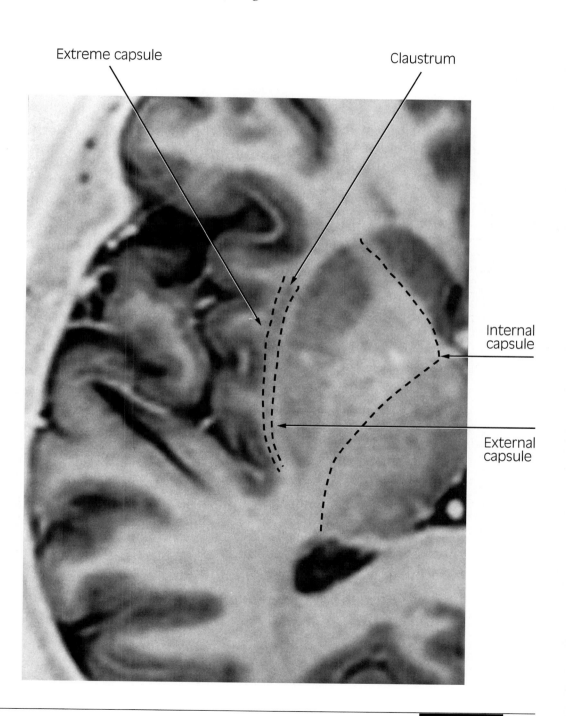

Extreme capsule

Claustrum

Internal capsule

External capsule

Figure **12.2**

Internal capsule, axial view, magnified.

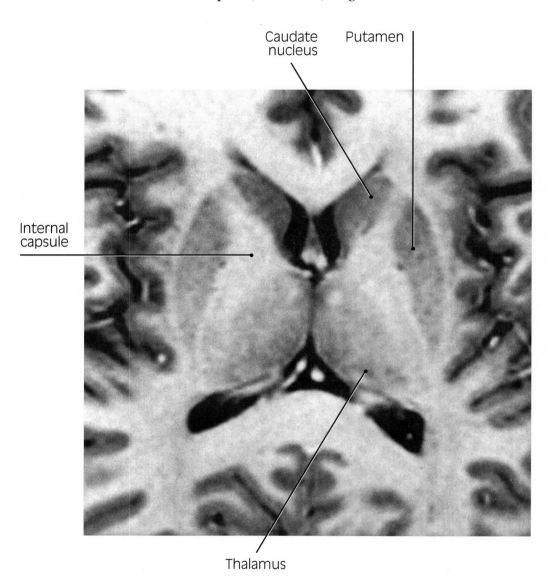

Caudate nucleus

Putamen

Internal capsule

Thalamus

Figure **12.3**

Internal capsule and gray matter nuclei,
axial view, magnified.

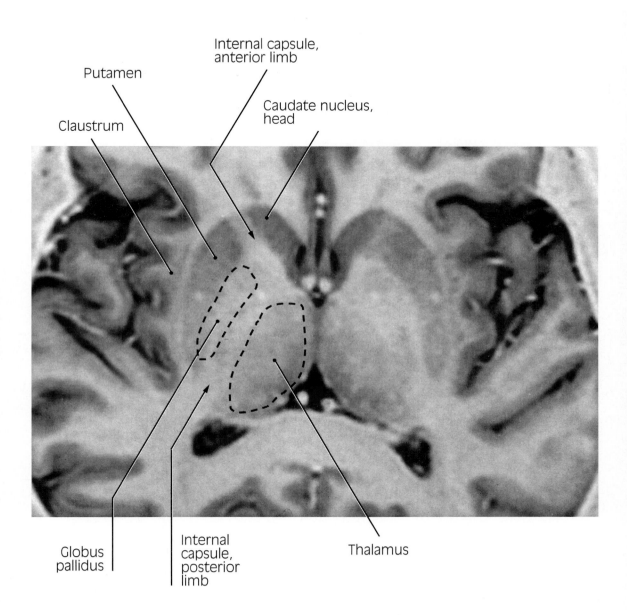

Internal capsule,
anterior limb

Putamen

Caudate nucleus,
head

Claustrum

Globus
pallidus

Internal
capsule,
posterior
limb

Thalamus

## Parts of the Internal Capsule

(Figure **12.4**)

| Parts | Location | Ascending Fibers | Descending Fibers |
|---|---|---|---|
| Anterior limb | Between caudate nucleus head and putamen | Anterior thalamic radiation | Auditory radiation Frontopontine |
| Genu | Between anterior and posterior limbs | Anterior superior thalamic radiation | Corticonuclear |
| Posterior limb | Between thalamus and lentiform nucleus | Superior thalamic radiation | Corticospinal Corticopontine Corticorubral |
| Retrolentiform | Behind lentiform nucleus | Globus pallidus to subthalamic nucleus | Parietopontine Occipitopontine Occipital cortex to superior colliculus and pretectal region |
| Sublentiform | Below lentiform nucleus | Posterior thalamic, mainly optic radiation | Parietopontine Occipitopontine Temporal lobe and thalamus |

## Orientation of the Body Parts in the Internal Capsule

(Figure **12.5**)

Figure **12.4**

Internal capsule, parts, axial view, magnified.

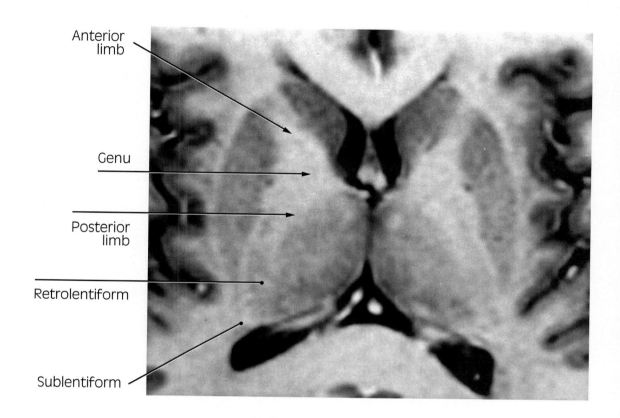

Anterior
limb

Genu

Posterior
limb

Retrolentiform

Sublentiform

Figure **12.5**

Internal capsule, body orientation, axial view, magnified.

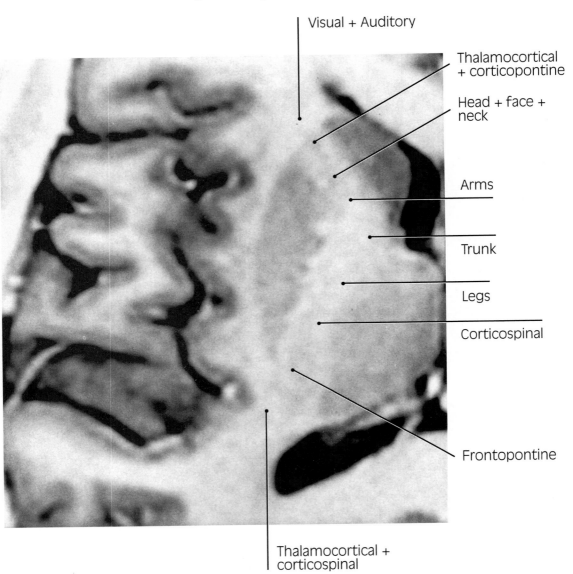

Visual + Auditory

Thalamocortical + corticopontine

Head + face + neck

Arms

Trunk

Legs

Corticospinal

Frontopontine

Thalamocortical + corticospinal

# CHAPTER 13

# Gray Matter Nuclei

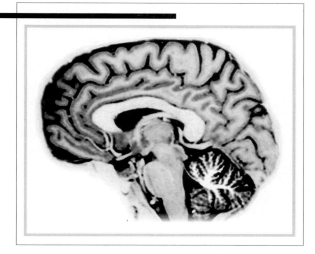

In the supratentorial space:   Corpus striatum

Claustrum

Amygdaloid body or amygdala

Thalami

In the infratentorial space:   Dentate

Emboliform

Fastigeal

Globose

## Corpus Striatum

(Figures **13.1** to **13.4**)

Location:   Between the insula and the midline

Nuclei:   Caudate

Lentiform:  Medial part: Globus pallidus

Lateral part: Putamen

Striated bands of gray matter interconnect the caudate and the lentiform nuclei (Figure **13.5**).

## Morphologic Divisions of Corpus Striatum

| Divisions | Synonym | Generation | Nuclei |
| --- | --- | --- | --- |
| Neostriatum | Striatum | Recent development | Caudate Putamen |
| Paleostriatum | Pallidum | Older primitive | Globus pallidus |

Figure **13.1**

Gray matter nuclei, sagittal view, magnified.

Caudate nucleus, head

Lateral ventricle

Internal capsule

Thalamus

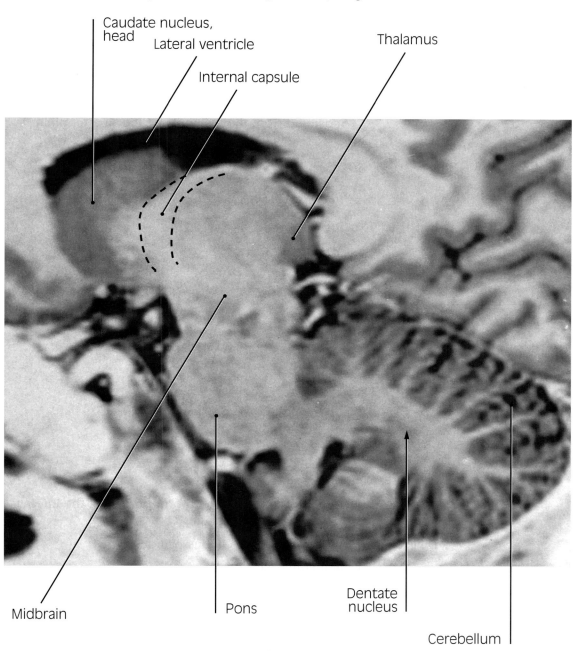

Midbrain

Pons

Dentate nucleus

Cerebellum

## FUNCTIONAL CONSIDERATIONS

The corpus striatum is involved with coordination of smooth voluntary and automatic associated movements.

- Parkinson's disease:

    Depletion of dopamine in the caudate nucleus and putamen

    Results:   Hypokinesia

    Bradykinesia

    Cogwheel rigidity

    Pill-rolling resting tremors

- Huntington's disease or chorea:

    Severe degeneration of the cholinergic and GABA-ergic neurons in the caudate nucleus and putamen

    Results:   Choreiform movements

    Progressive dementia

    Hydrocephalus ex vacuo

- Hepatolenticular degeneration or Wilson's disease:

    Lesions in the lentiform nuclei and liver due to a defect in copper metabolism

    Results:   Tremor

    Rigidity

    Choreiform or athetotic movements

Figure **13.1**

Gray matter nuclei, sagittal view, magnified.

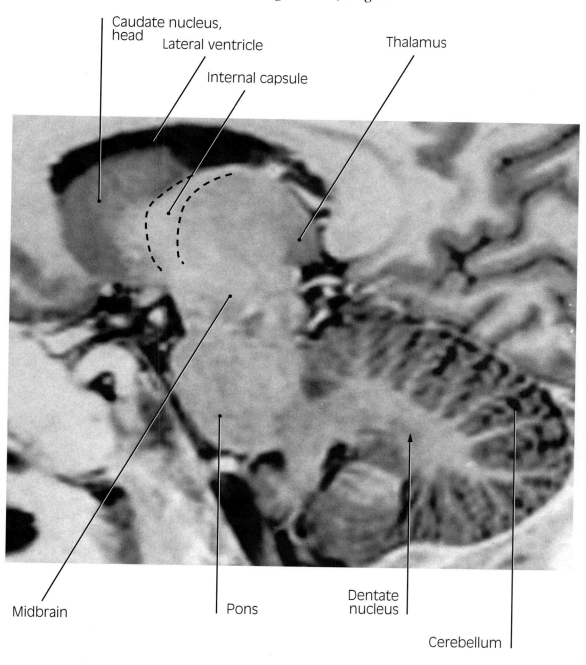

Caudate nucleus, head

Lateral ventricle

Internal capsule

Thalamus

Midbrain

Pons

Dentate nucleus

Cerebellum

## Caudate Nucleus

Shape:   C-shaped or comma-shaped

Parts:   Head: Forms the floor of the anterior horn of the lateral ventricle and the medial wall of the anterior limb of the internal capsule.

Body: Forms the floor of the central part of the lateral ventricle. Located medial to the posterior limb of the internal capsule.

Separated from the thalamus by the stria terminalis and the thalamostriate vein.

Tail: Forms the roof of the inferior horn of the lateral ventricle and ends by joining the amygdaloid body at the temporal pole.

## Lentiform Nuclei

Shape:   Biconvex or lens-shaped

Surfaces:   Medial: Convex

Related to: Internal capsule

Caudate nucleus

Thalamus

Lateral: Convex

Related to: External capsule

Claustrum

Extreme capsule

Insula

Inferior: Pointed

Related to: Sublentiform portion of the internal capsule

Divisions:   Medial smaller part: Globus pallidus

Lateral larger part: Putamen

Figure **13.2**

Gray matter nuclei, sagittal view, magnified.

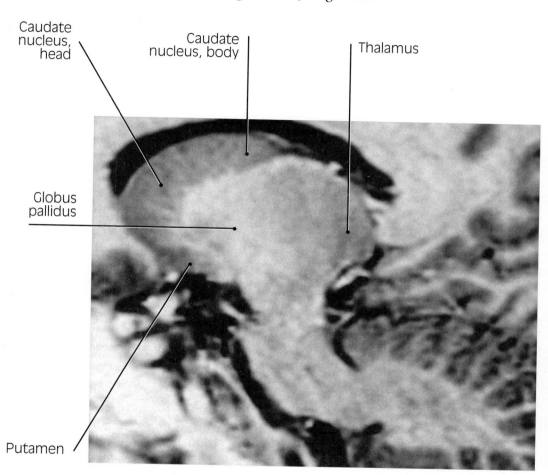

Caudate
nucleus,
head

Caudate
nucleus, body

Thalamus

Globus
pallidus

Putamen

## FUNCTIONAL CONSIDERATIONS

The corpus striatum is involved with coordination of smooth voluntary and automatic associated movements.

- Parkinson's disease:

  Depletion of dopamine in the caudate nucleus and putamen

  Results:  Hypokinesia

  Bradykinesia

  Cogwheel rigidity

  Pill-rolling resting tremors

- Huntington's disease or chorea:

  Severe degeneration of the cholinergic and GABA-ergic neurons in the caudate nucleus and putamen

  Results:  Choreiform movements

  Progressive dementia

  Hydrocephalus ex vacuo

- Hepatolenticular degeneration or Wilson's disease:

  Lesions in the lentiform nuclei and liver due to a defect in copper metabolism

  Results:  Tremor

  Rigidity

  Choreiform or athetotic movements

Figure **13.3**

Gray matter nuclei and internal capsule, sagittal view, magnified.

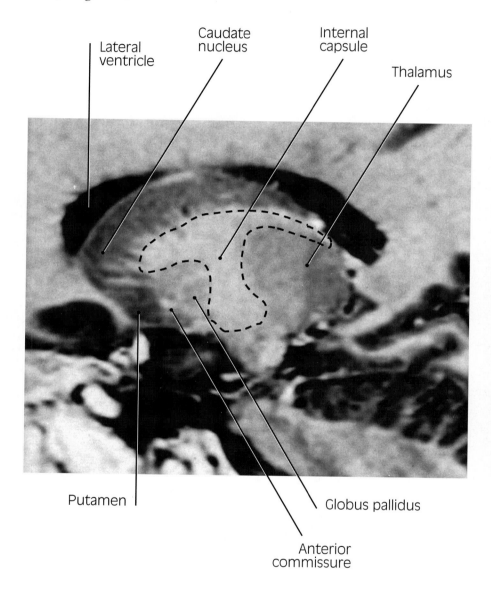

Lateral ventricle

Caudate nucleus

Internal capsule

Thalamus

Putamen

Globus pallidus

Anterior commissure

Figure **13.4**

Gray matter nuclei, axial view, magnified.

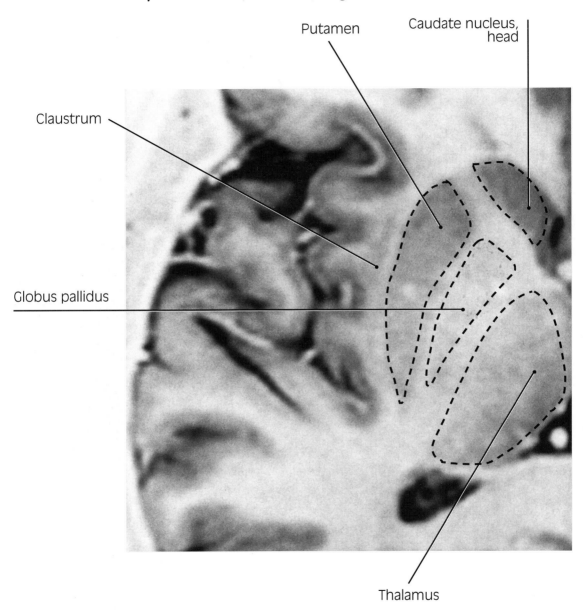

Putamen

Caudate nucleus, head

Claustrum

Globus pallidus

Thalamus

Figure **13.5**

Corpus striatum, coronal view.

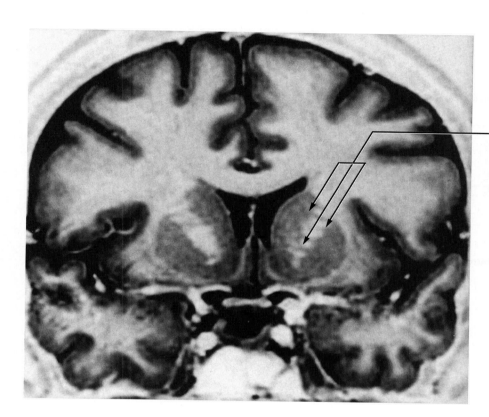

Striated
bands of
corpus
striatum

## Claustrum

(Figure **13.6**)

**Shape:**   Saucer-shaped

**Location:**   Between the putamen and the insula

**Ends:**   Inferiorly by continuing with the anterior perforated substance

## Amygdaloid Body or Amygdala

**Location:**   Nuclear mass in the temporal lobe, anterosuperior to the inferior horn of the lateral ventricle and underlying the parahippocampal uncus

### FUNCTIONAL CONSIDERATION

Part of the limbic system (discussed with the limbic system)

## Thalamic Nuclei

(Discussed with diencephalon)

Figure **13.6**

Gray matter nuclei, coronal view, magnified.

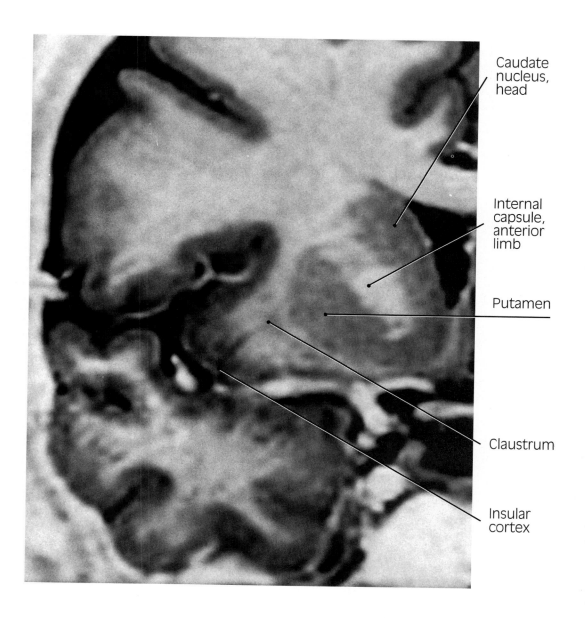

Caudate nucleus, head

Internal capsule, anterior limb

Putamen

Claustrum

Insular cortex

# CHAPTER 14

# Ventricular System

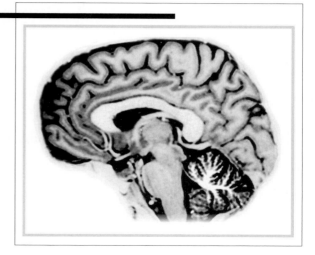

The ventricular system consists of four fluid-filled communicating cavities, as follows:

Lateral ventricles

Third ventricle

Fourth ventricle

## Flow of the Ventricular System

From choroid plexus in the floor of the lateral ventricle
↓
Interventricular foramen of Monro
↓
Third ventricle
↓
Cerebral aqueduct of Sylvius (Iter)
↓
Fourth ventricle
↓
Foramina of Magendie and Luschka
↓
To brain cisterns and cervical subarachnoid space
↓
Intrathecal spinal compartment
↓
Percolates over the convexity of the hemispheres
↓
Resorbed by arachnoid villi into the intravascular space

## Lateral Ventricles

(Figures **14.1** to **14.9**)

Location:   Two cavities in the telencephalon or one in each
cerebral hemisphere

Figure **14.1**

Lateral ventricles, axial view, magnified.

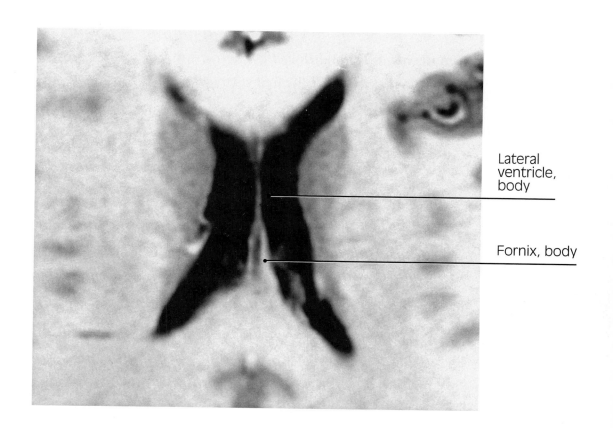

Lateral
ventricle,
body

Fornix, body

Parts:  Anterior or frontal horns

Body

Trigone

Posterior or occipital horns

Inferior or temporal horns

## Anterior or Frontal Horns

Location:  In front of the interventricular foramen

Shape:  Triangular

Direction:  Forward, lateral, and downward

Relationships:  Anterior: Posterior surface of genu and rostrum of the corpus callosum

Superior: Posterior surface of genu of the corpus callosum

Roof: Anterior part of body of the corpus callosum

Medial: Septum pellucidum and septal nuclei

Lateral: Head of the caudate nucleus

## Body of the Lateral Ventricle

Location:  From the interventricular foramen to the splenium of the corpus callosum

Relationships:  Roof: Undersurface of the corpus callosum

Medial: Septum pellucidum

Body of fornix

Lateral: Body of the caudate nucleus

Floor: Body of the caudate nucleus

Stria terminalis

Thalamostriate vein

Lateral walls of the upper thalamus

## Trigone of the Lateral Ventricle

Location:  At the junction of the body, occipital horn, and temporal horn of the lateral ventricle

Contents:  Glomus, a large tuft of the choroid plexus

Relationships:  Medial: Hippocampus

Lateral: Optic radiation

Figure **14.2**

Lateral ventricles, axial view, magnified.

Cavum septum
pellucidum

Lateral
ventricle,
frontal
horn

Fornix

Third
ventricle

Lateral
ventricle,
atrium

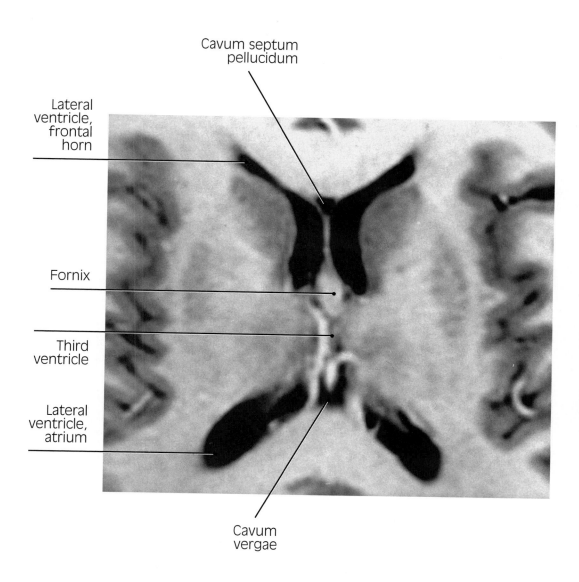

Cavum
vergae

## Posterior or Occipital Horns

Location:   Behind the splenium of the corpus callosum, extending in the occipital lobes

Direction:   Backward and medially

Relationships:   Superior, lateral, and inferior: Optic radiation

Medial: Calcar avis and calcarine cortex

> **N O T E**   The posterior horns are variable in size and may be absent. They also lack choroid plexus.

## Inferior or Temporal Horns

The largest part or horn of the lateral ventricle

Location:   In the temporal lobe

Relationships:   Roof: Tail of the caudate nucleus

Anterior: Amygdala

Medial: Hippocampus

Fimbria

Choroidal fissure

Lateral: Association fibers anteriorly

Meyer's loop of optic radiation posteriorly

> **N O T E**   The choroid plexus in the inferior horns lies between the stria terminalis and the fimbria.

## Interventricular Foramen of Monro

It connects the lateral ventricles to the third ventricle.

Contents:   Choroid plexus

Thalamostriate vein

Internal cerebral vein

Relationships:   Anterosuperior: Fornix

Anterolateral: Head of the caudate nucleus

Posterior: Massa intermedia with thalamic tubercle

Lateral: Genu of the internal capsule

Figure **14.3**

Third ventricle, axial view, magnified.

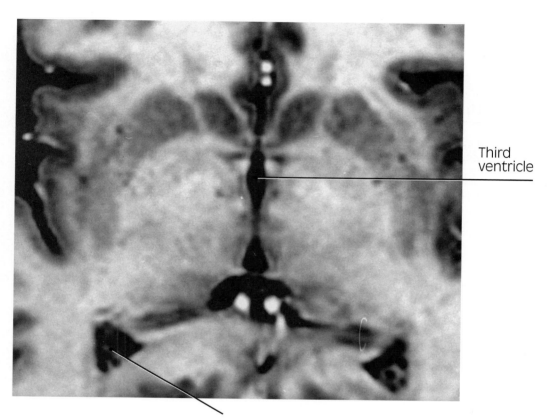

Third
ventricle

Lateral ventricle,
choroid plexus

Figure **14.4**

Lateral and third ventricles, axial view, magnified.

Frontal horn

Fornix

Third ventricle

Cavum of
velum
interpositum

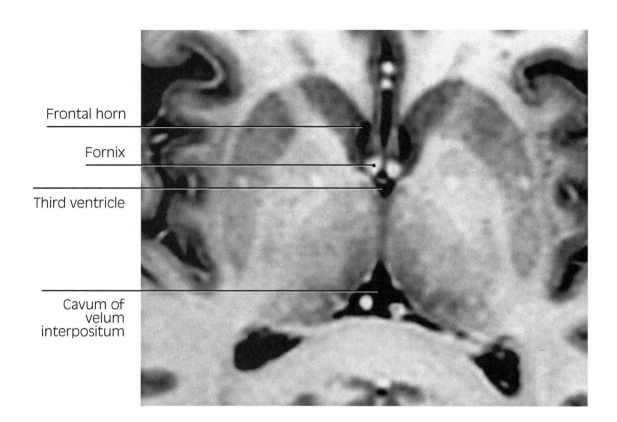

Figure **14.5**

Lateral ventricles, temporal horn, axial view.

Temporal horn

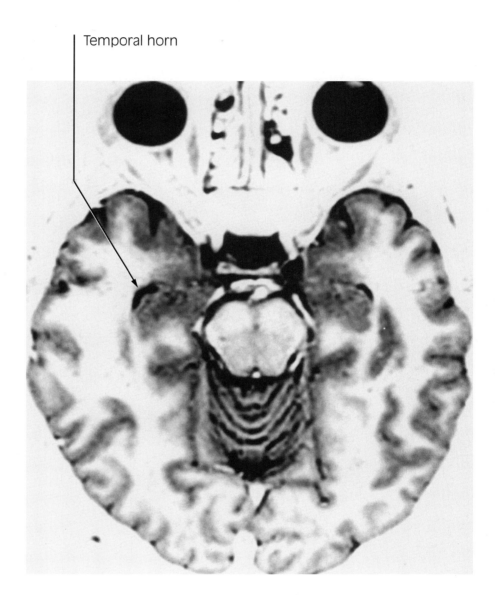

Figure **14.6**

Lateral ventricles, temporal horn, axial view.

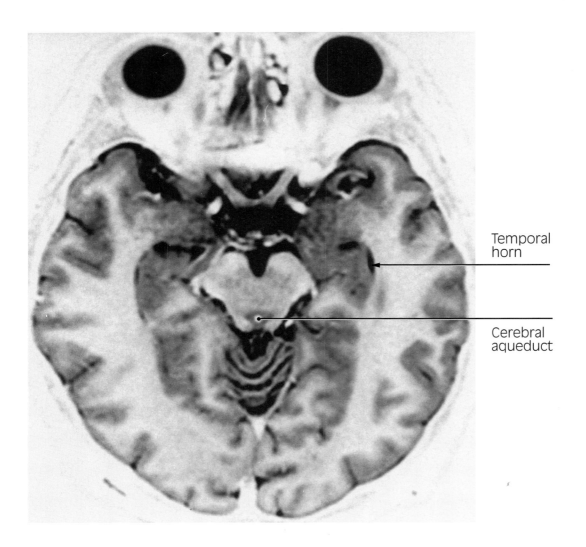

Temporal horn

Cerebral aqueduct

Figure **14.7**

Lateral ventricles, posterior horn, sagittal view.

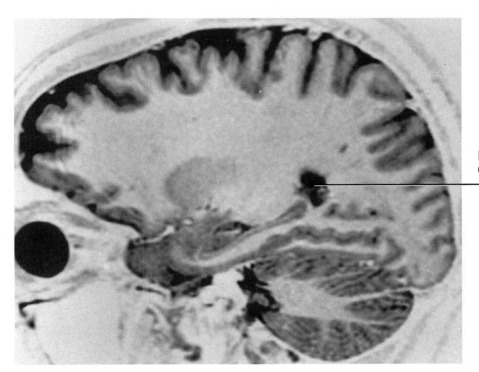

Posterior or
occipital horn

Figure **14.8**

Lateral ventricles, posterior horn, axial view.

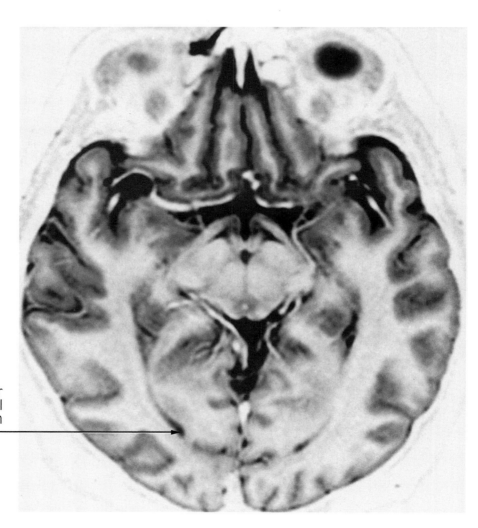

Posterior or
occipital
horn

Figure **14.9**

Lateral ventricle, axial view, magnified.

Lateral
ventricle,
temporal
horn

Cerebral
aqueduct

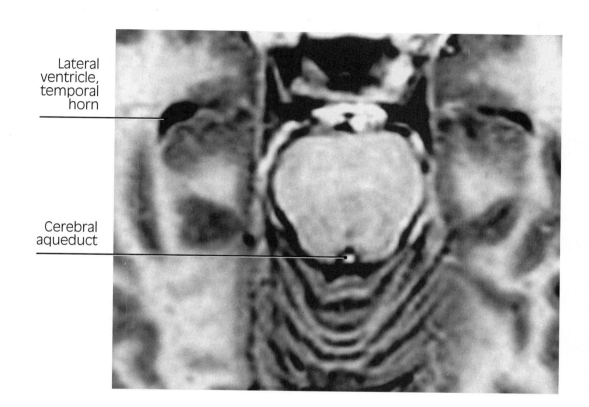

# Third Ventricle

(Figures **14.10** and **14.11**)

See also Figure **14.3.**

**Location:**   Between the thalamus and hypothalamus, in the diencephalon

**Appearance:**   As a median cleft

**Recesses:**   Suprapineal

Pineal

Infundibular

Optic

Figure **14.10**

Foramen of Monro, axial view, magnified.

Lateral ventricle,
frontal horn

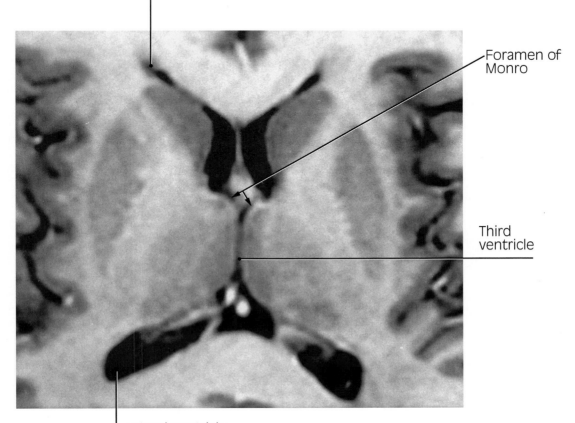

Foramen of
Monro

Third
ventricle

Lateral ventricle,
atrium

Relationships:    Anterior: Lamina terminalis

Anterior commissure

Columns of fornix

Posterosuperior: Pineal recess

Posterior commissure

Posteroinferior: Tegmentum

Roof: Stria medullaris with interconnecting choroid

Floor: Hypothalamic structures

Optic chiasm

Tuber cinereum

Infundibular stalk

Mamillary body

Posterior perforated substance

Tegmentum

Medial: Massa intermedia

Lateral: Medial surface of the thalamus

Hypothalamus with its sulcus

Figure **14.11**

Third ventricle, sagittal view, magnified.

Cavum septum
pellucidum

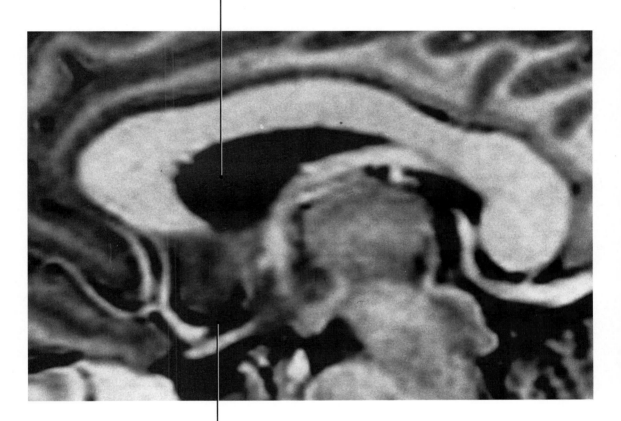

Third
ventricle

## Cerebral Aqueduct of Sylvius

(Figures **14.12** and **14.13**)

Location: Between the third and fourth ventricles, in the mesencephalon

Relationships:  Anterior: Red nucleus

Brachium conjunctivum

Roof: Posterior commissure

Tectal or quadrigeminal plate

Floor: Oculomotor nerve nucleus

Trochlear nerve nucleus

Medial longitudinal fasciculus

## Fourth Ventricle

(Figures **14.14** to **14.19**)

Location: Cavity of the hindbrain, between the pons and medulla in front and the cerebellum behind

Shape: Tent-shaped

| *Part* | *Formation by* |
|---|---|
| Apex or extreme roof | Superior medullary velum |
| Superior lateral part | Superior cerebellar peduncles<br>Tela choroidea and choroid plexus |
| Middle part | Lateral walls: Middle cerebellar peduncle<br>Inferior cerebellar peduncle<br>Roof: Vermis<br>Floor: Nuclei: Abducens, facial, vestibular<br>Medial longitudinal fasciculus |
| Inferior part or floor<br>(also called the rhomboid fossa) | Roof: Inferior medullary velum<br>Median foramen of magendie<br>Nodulus of vermis |
| | Floor: Posterior pons and medulla<br>Vagal and hypoglossal nuclei<br>Medial longitudinal fasciculus |
| Obex (extreme caudal point of the fourth ventricle) | Lateral wall: Area postrema<br>Gracile nuclei |
| | Floor: Hypoglossal nuclei<br>Medial longitudinal fasciculus |

Figure **14.12**

Cerebral aqueduct, sagittal view, magnified.

Lateral ventricle/ cavum septum pellucidum

Foramen of Monro

Third ventricle

Cerebral aqueduct

Fourth ventricle

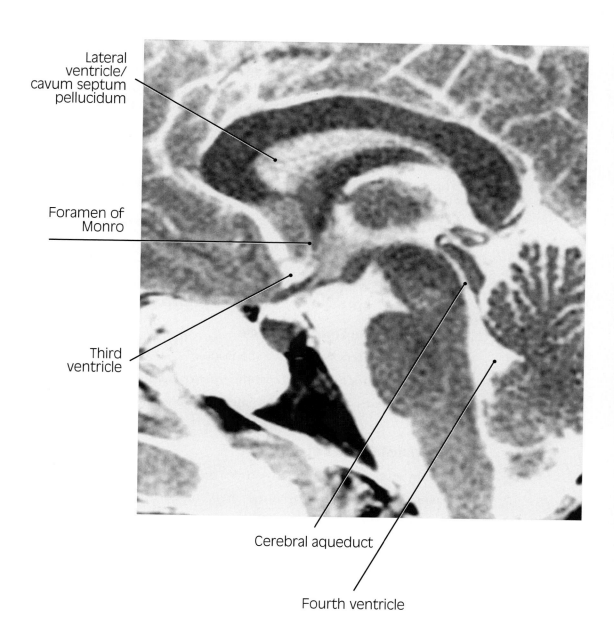

> **NOTE** The median sulcus divides the floor of the fourth ventricle into the right and left halves.
>
> In the superior portion of each half, the structures from medial to lateral are the facial colliculus, superior fovea, vestibular area, and stria medullaris.
>
> The two important triangles in the inferior anterior portion are the hypoglossal and the vagal triangle medially and laterally, respectively. In the inferior posterior portion, the important structures are the area postrema and the obex.

## Communications of the Fourth Ventricle

Superiorly:   With the third ventricle through the aqueduct of Sylvius

Inferiorly:   With the central canal of the medulla and spinal cord

Dorsally:   With the subarachnoid space of the cisterna magna through the median aperture or foramen of Magendie

Either side:   With the subarachnoid space through the lateral apertures or foramina of Luschka

## Recesses of the Fourth Ventricle

Median dorsal recess:   Above the nodule

Lateral dorsal recesses:   Above the inferior medullary velum

Lateral recesses:   Between the inferior cerebellar peduncle and the flocculus

## Associated Cavities of the Brain

Cavum septi pellucidi:   Between leaves of the septum pellucidum

Cavum vergae:   Posterior to the interventricular foramen

Cavum of velum interpositum:   Rostral extension of the quadrigeminal cistern

Figure **14.13**

Cerebral aqueduct, axial view, magnified.

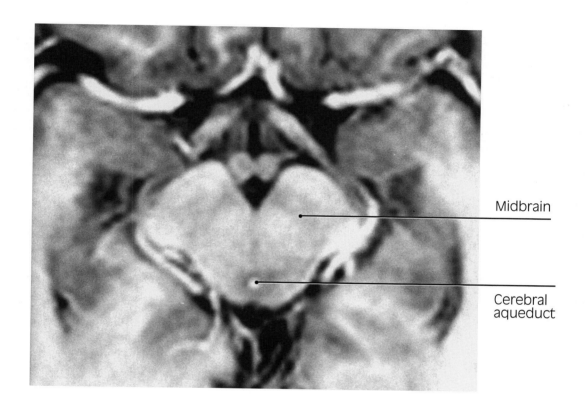

Midbrain

Cerebral
aqueduct

## Cerebrospinal Fluid (CSF) Characteristics

Clear, acellular fluid in the subarachnoid space and in the ventricles

**Production:**   500 ml per day

**Formation:**   By the choroid plexus

**Composition:**   pH 7.5; specific gravity 1.007

Glucose 65 mg/dl

Total proteins 15–50 mg/dl in the lumbar cistern

Lymphocytes less than five per ml

**Pressure:**   50–200 mm of water in the lumbar subarachnoid space in the lateral recumbent position

**PRACTICAL POINTS**

Asymmetry of the lateral ventricles may be a normal variant because of a plane of the image. However, such an appearance may be due to a block of the interventricular foramen or to an increased mass effect or brain loss.

Local tumors or developmental defects easily obstruct the narrow tract of the third ventricle.

Aqueductal stenosis results in hydrocephalus.

Injury of the vagal triangle in the fourth ventricle is usually fatal.

Infratentorial tumors block the lateral and median foramina, resulting in a marked increase in intracranial pressure.

Figure **14.14**

Fourth ventricle, sagittal view, magnified.

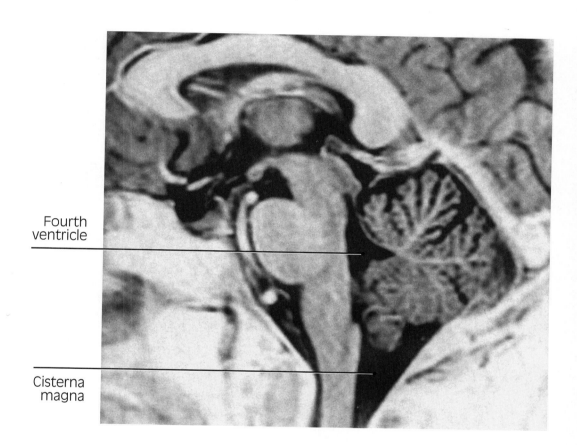

Fourth
ventricle

Cisterna
magna

Figure **14.15**

Fourth ventricle, sagittal view, magnified.

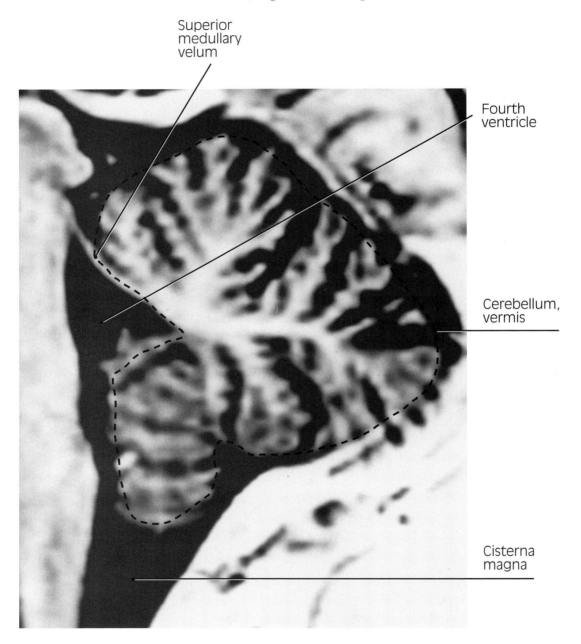

Superior medullary velum

Fourth ventricle

Cerebellum, vermis

Cisterna magna

Figure **14.16**

Fourth ventricle, axial view, magnified.

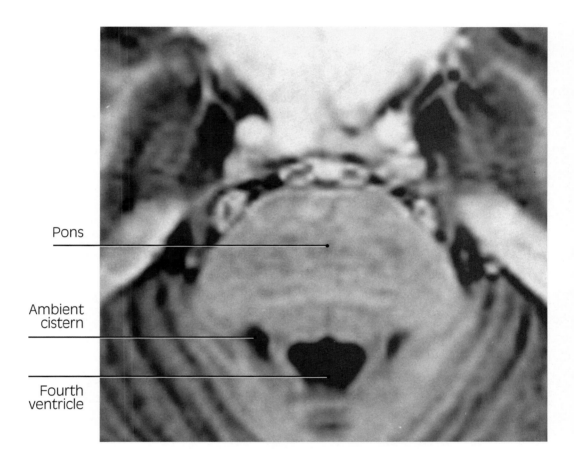

Pons

Ambient
cistern

Fourth
ventricle

Figure **14.17**

Fourth ventricle, coronal view, magnified.

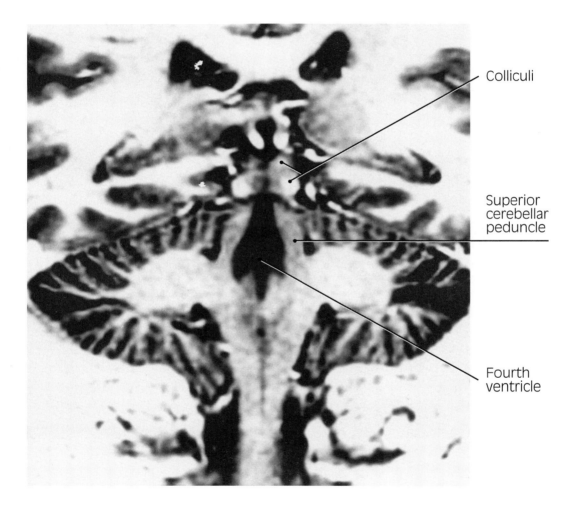

Colliculi

Superior
cerebellar
peduncle

Fourth
ventricle

Figure **14.18**

Fourth ventricle, coronal view, magnified.

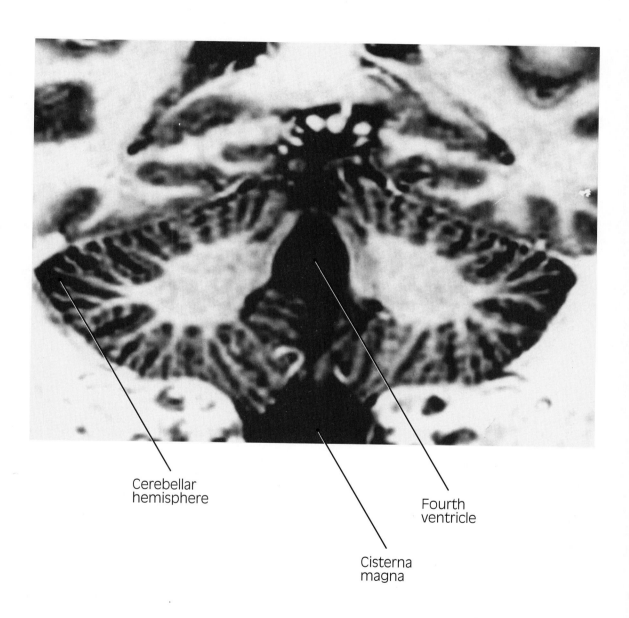

Cerebellar
hemisphere

Fourth
ventricle

Cisterna
magna

Figure **14.19**

Fourth ventricle, coronal view, magnified.

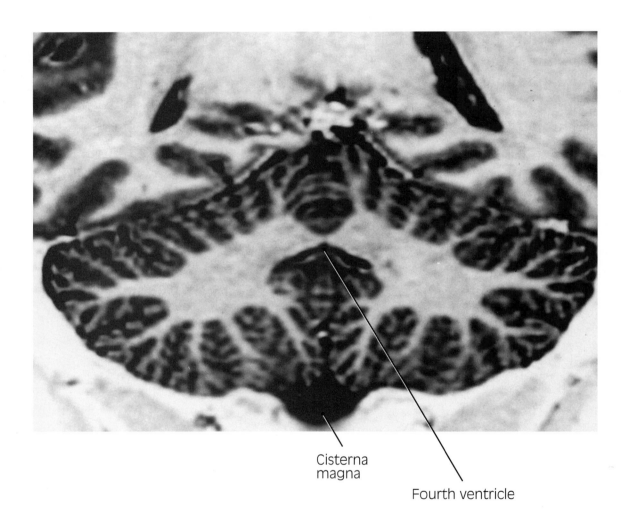

Cisterna
magna

Fourth ventricle

# CHAPTER 15

# Cisternal Anatomy

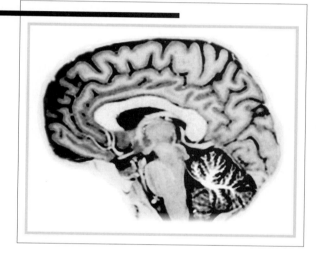

(Figures **15.1** to **15.20**)

| Cisterns | Location | Contents |
|---|---|---|
| Subarachnoid space over cerebral cortex | Hemispheric surface | Cerebral veins and arteries |
| Interhemispheric | Between the hemispheres, either side of falx | Anterior cerebral artery Anterior communicating artery |
| Cistern of ACA | Above corpus callosum | Anterior cerebral artery |
| Cistern of lamina terminalis | Anterior to lamina terminalis | Anterior cerebral artery |
| Cistern of velum interpositum | Above third ventricle | Internal cerebral vein Vein of Galen |
| Callosal | Along superior surface of the corpus callosum | Pericallosal artery |
| Insular | Over insular lobe | Middle cerebral artery and branches |
| Lateral sylvian | In sylvian fissure | Middle cerebral artery and branches |
| Suprasellar, pentagonal | Above pituitary | Optic chiasm Internal carotid artery and bifurcation Pituitary stalk Arteries:    Posterior communicating    Arterior choroidal    Ophthalmic    Anterior perforating Veins:    Basal    Middle cerebral    Deep cerebral Nerves:    Optic    Oculomotor |
| Cistern of velum interpositum | Below fornix and above pulvinar | Choroidal arteries Internal cerebral vein |

| | | |
|---|---|---|
| Quadrigeminal | Behind quadrigeminal plate | Posterior cerebral artery<br>Posterior choroidal artery<br>Vein of Galen<br>Basal vein<br>Deep cerebral vein<br>Trochlear nerve<br>Pineal gland |
| Interpeduncular | Between cerebral peduncles, anterior to midbrain | Oculomotor nerve<br>Upper end of basilar artery |
| Ambient or crural | Around midbrain | Trochlear nerve<br>Posterior cerebral artery<br>Superior cerebellar artery<br>Optic tract |
| Retropulvinar | Behind thalamus | Posterolateral choroidal artery |
| Superior cerebellar | Above cerebellum<br>Below tentorium | Basal vein of Rosenthal<br>Vein of Galen |
| Prepontine | Anterior to pons | Basilar artery<br>Trigeminal nerve<br>Abducens nerve |
| Lateral pontine | Between temporal bone and brachium pontis | Trigeminal nerve |
| Cerebellopontine angle | Between pons and porus acusticus | Anteroinferior cerebellar artery<br>Facial nerve<br>Vestibulocochlear nerve |
| Premedullary | Between medulla and clivus | Vertebral arteries<br>Accessory nerve<br>Hypoglossal nerve |
| Lateral medullary | Lateral to medulla | Vertebral arteries<br>Glossopharyngeal nerve<br>Vagus nerve<br>Accessory nerve<br>Hypoglossal nerve |
| Circummedullary velum | Around medulla | Posteroinferior cerebellar artery |
| Cisterna magna | Posteroinferior to fourth ventricle | Posterior inferior cerebellar artery<br>Last four cranial nerves<br>Vertebral arteries<br>Tonsils |

Figure **15.1**

Subarachnoid space and interhemispheric cistern,
axial view.

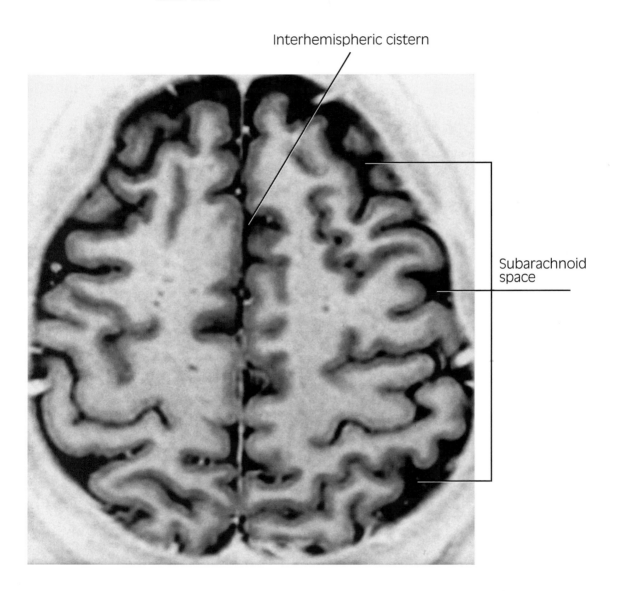

Figure **15.2**

Interhemispheric cistern, axial view.

Interhemispheric
cistern

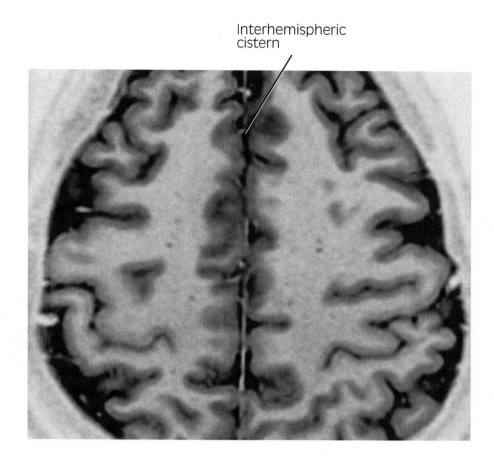

Figure **15.3**

Cistern of Aca, axial view.

Cistern of Aca

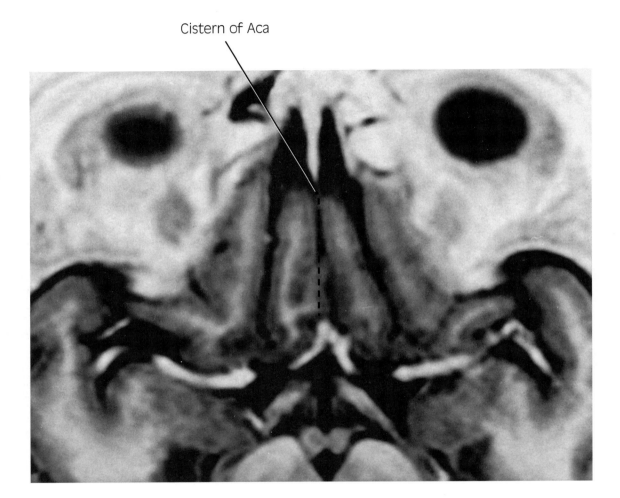

Figure **15.4**

Midline cisterns, sagittal view.

**Cisterns:**

Callosal      Lamina terminalis      Suprapineal

Hypothalamic

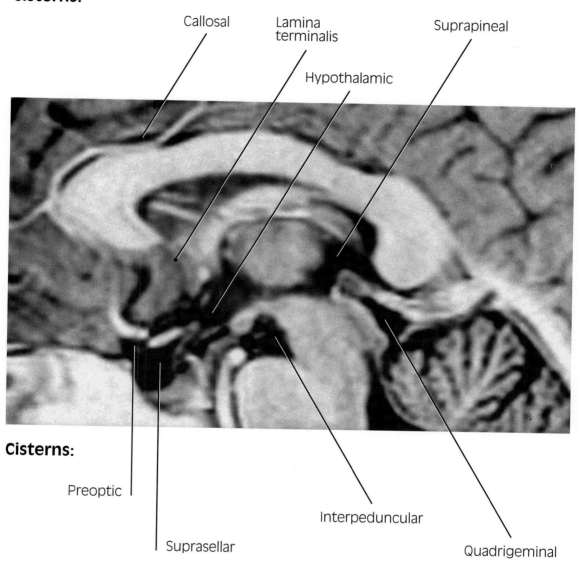

**Cisterns:**

Preoptic

Suprasellar

Interpeduncular

Quadrigeminal

Figure **15.5**

Insular cistern, axial view.

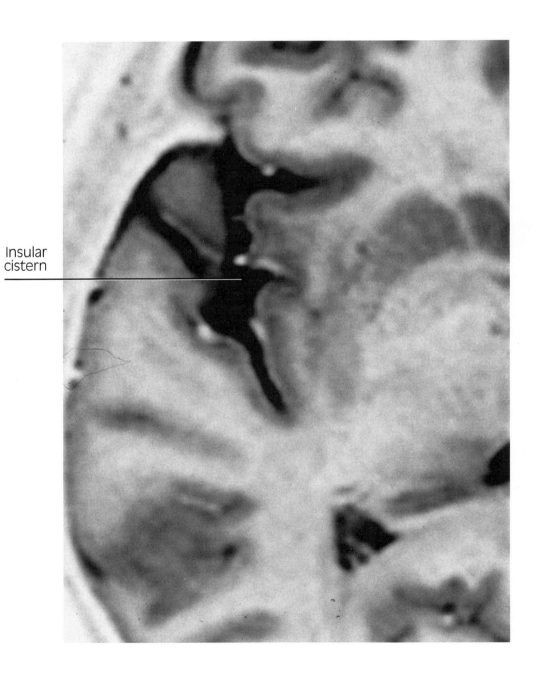

Insular
cistern

Figure **15.6**

Sylvian cistern, axial view.

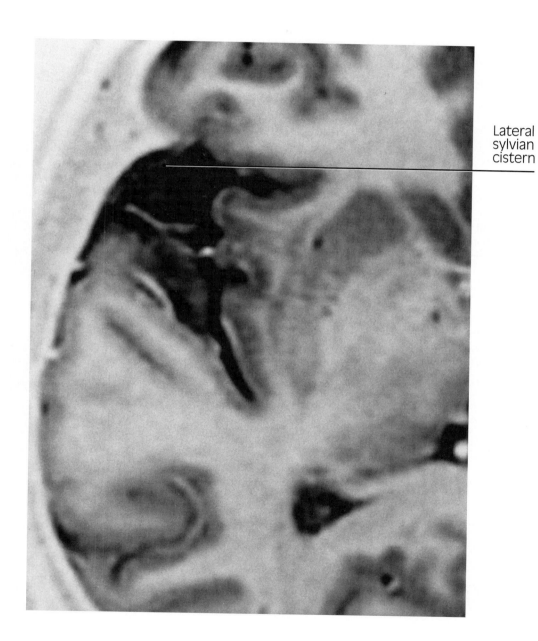

Lateral
sylvian
cistern

Figure **15.7**

Suprasellar cistern, coronal view.

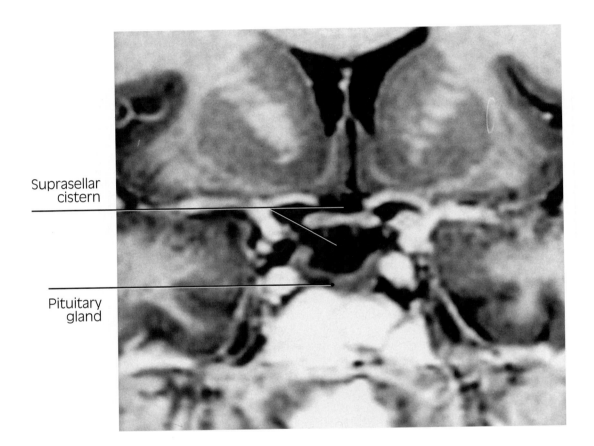

Suprasellar
cistern

Pituitary
gland

Figure **15.8**

Cisterns surrounding midbrain, axial view.

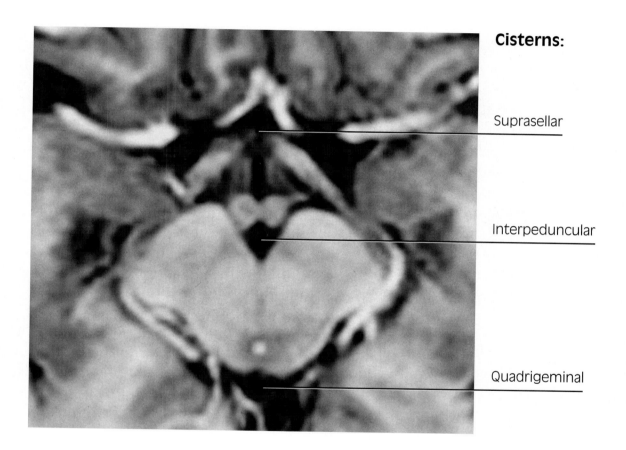

**Cisterns:**

Suprasellar

Interpeduncular

Quadrigeminal

Figure **15.9**

Midbrain cisterns, axial view.

Interpeduncular

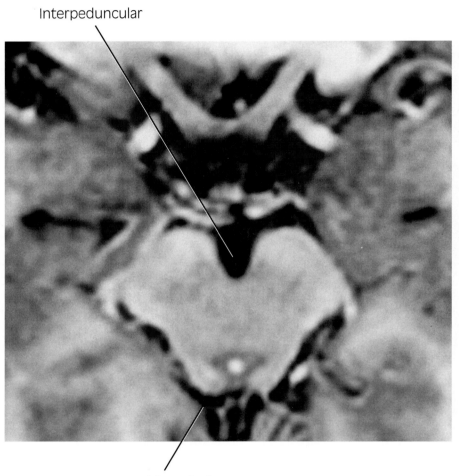

Quadrigeminal

Figure **15.10**

Retrosellar and ambient cisterns, axial view.

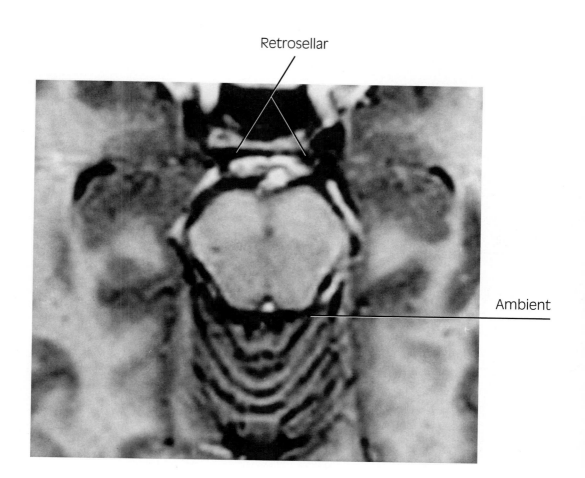

Figure **15.11**

Ambient cistern, axial view.

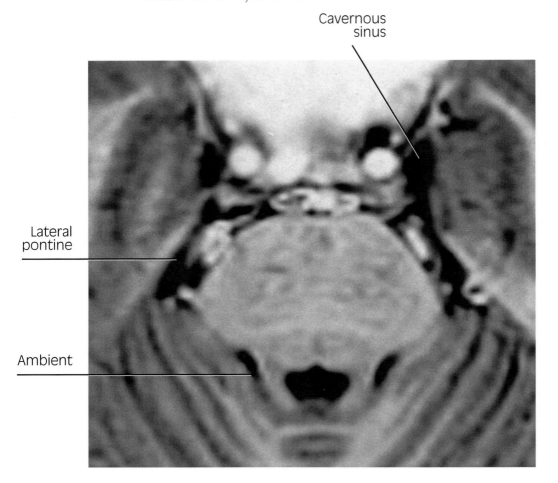

Cavernous
sinus

Lateral
pontine

Ambient

Figure **15.12**

Retropulvinar cistern, sagittal view.

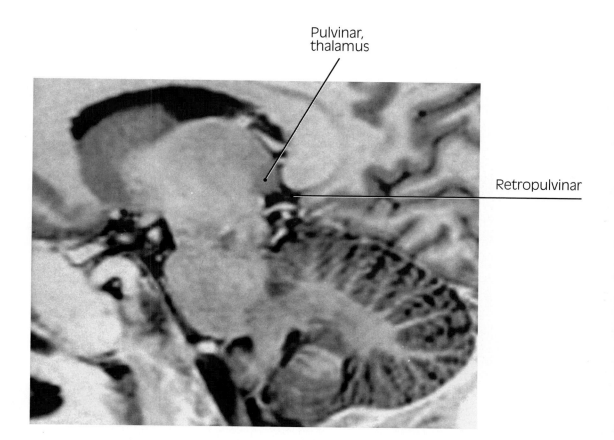

Figure **15.13**

Superior cerebellar cistern, coronal view.

Superior
cerebellar

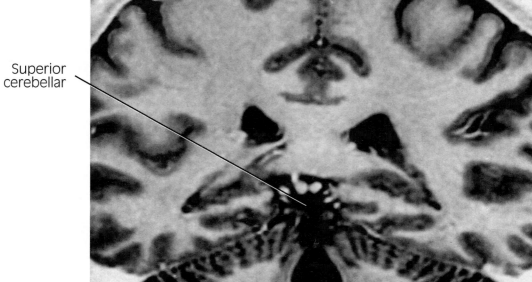

Figure **15.14**

Sellar, pontine, and medullary cisterns, sagittal view.

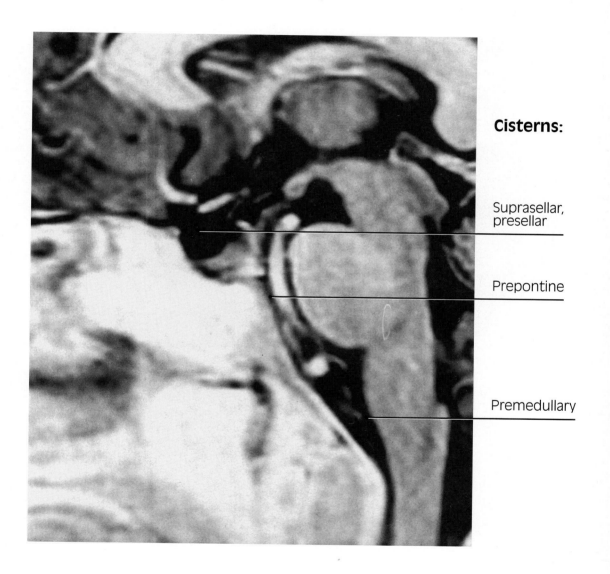

**Cisterns:**

Suprasellar, presellar

Prepontine

Premedullary

Figure **15.15**

Cerebellopontine angle cistern, axial view.

Cerebellopontine
angle cistern

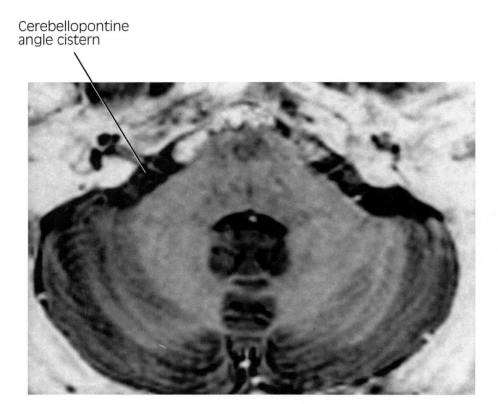

Figure **15.16**

Lateral pontine and medullary cisterns, coronal view, magnified.

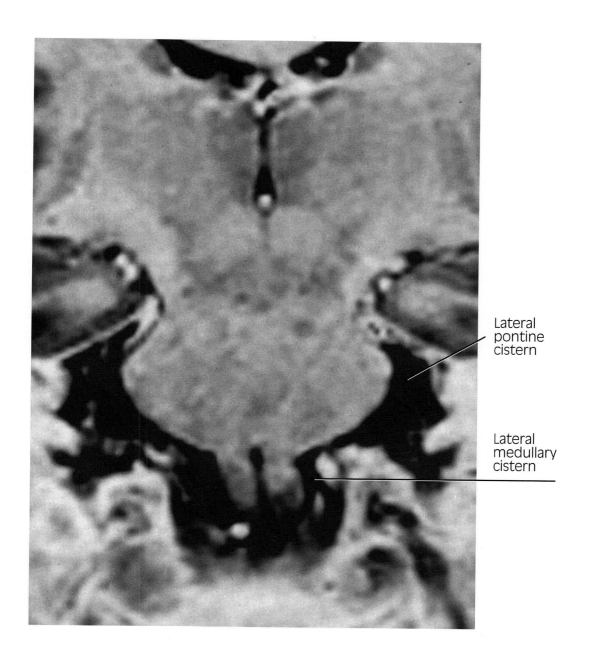

Lateral
pontine
cistern

Lateral
medullary
cistern

Figure **15.17**

Lateral medullary cistern, coronal view, magnified.

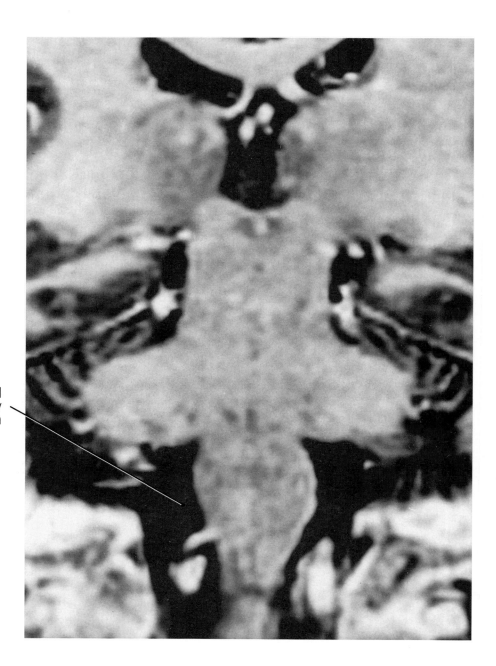

Lateral
medullary
cistern

Figure **15.18**

Medullary cisterns, axial view.

Paramedullary or
circummedullary

Premedullary

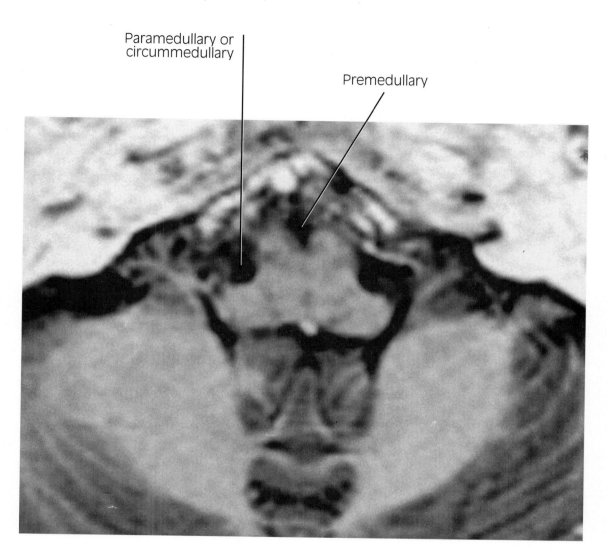

Figure **15.19**

Medullary cisterns, axial view.

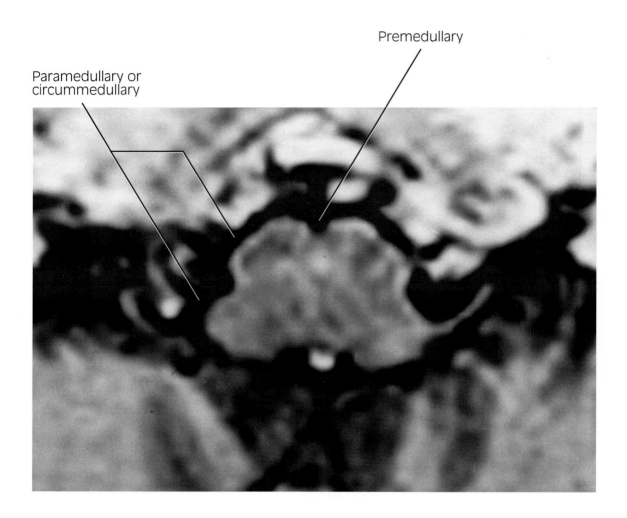

Premedullary

Paramedullary or
circummedullary

Figure **15.20**

Cisterna magna, sagittal view.

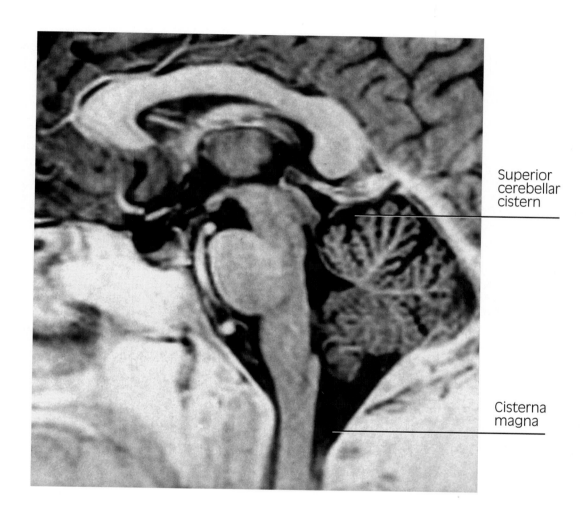

Superior
cerebellar
cistern

Cisterna
magna

# CHAPTER 16

# Cranial Nerves
## (Groups of Two and Four)

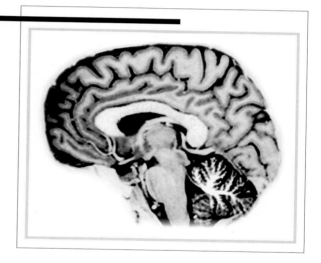

## Above Midbrain

### First Cranial Nerve: Olfactory
(Figures **16.1** to **16.5**)

Demonstration:     Olfactory bulbs along the medial and inferior
                    portions of the anterior cranial fossa

Supply:     Sensory: Olfactory epithelium of superior nasal cavity

Figure **16.1**

Olfactory nerve, sagittal view.

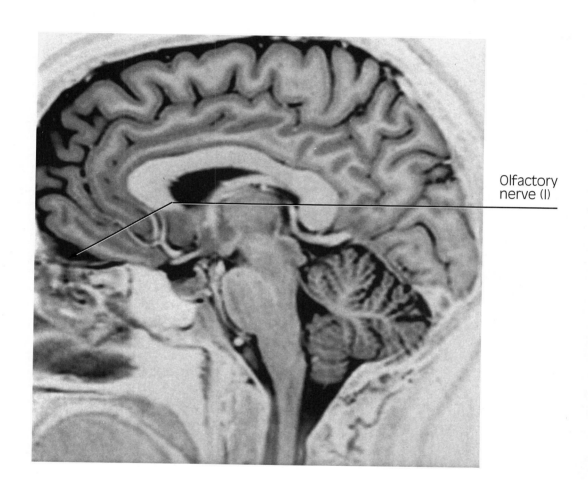

Olfactory
nerve (I)

Figure **16.2**

Olfactory cranial nerve, sagittal view, magnified.

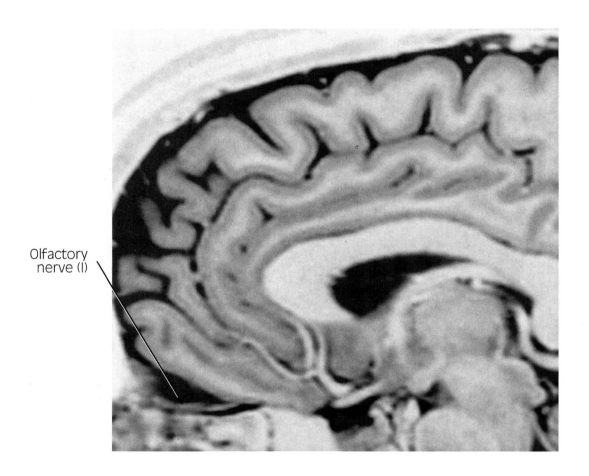

Olfactory
nerve (I)

Figure **16.3**

Olfactory cranial nerve, axial view, magnified.

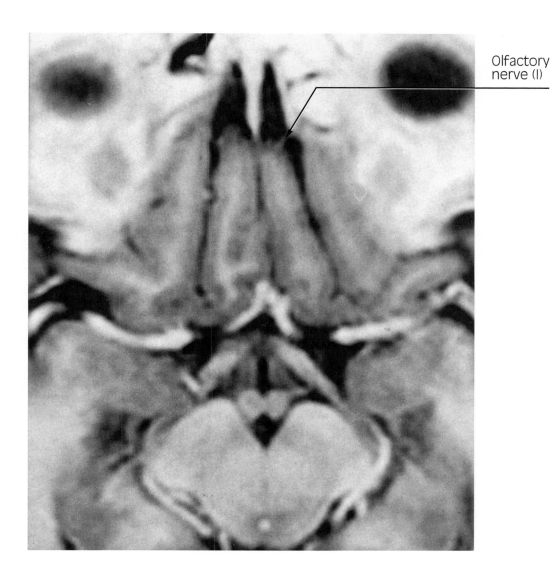

Olfactory nerve (I)

Figure **16.4**

Olfactory cranial nerve, coronal view, magnified.

Olfactory
nerve (I)

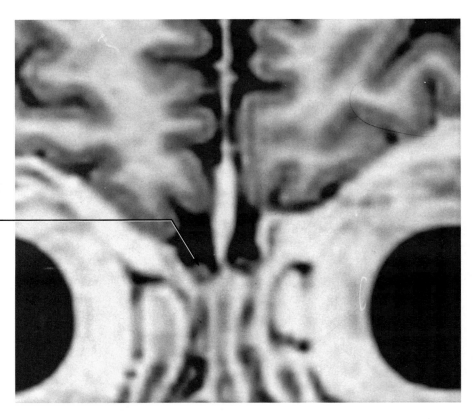

Figure **16.5**

Olfactory cranial nerve, coronal view, magnified.

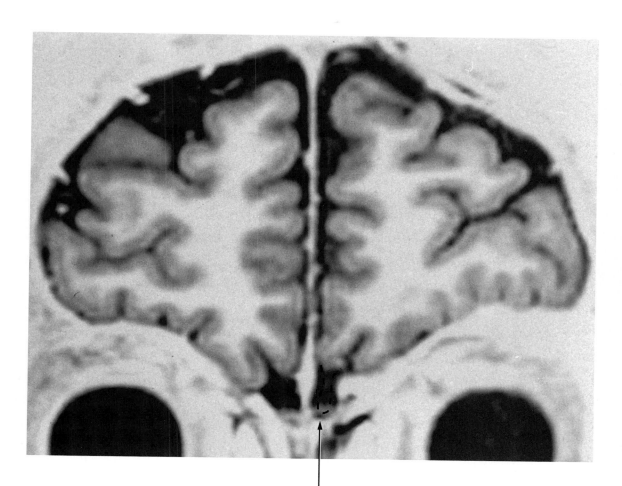

Olfactory
nerve (I)

## Second Cranial Nerve: Optic
(Figures **16.6** to **16.12**)

Demonstration:   In the center of the orbit, behind the globe; connection to lateral geniculate body

Supply:   Sensory: Retina

Figure **16.6**

Optic nerve, coronal view, magnified.

**Muscles:**

Superior oblique

Superior rectus

Medial rectus

Lateral rectus

Inferior rectus and oblique complex

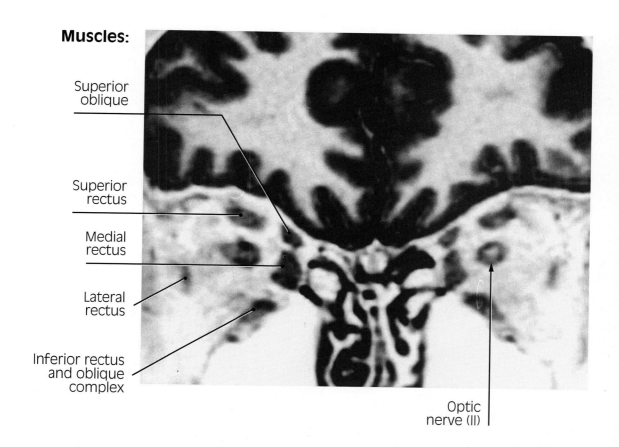

Optic nerve (II)

Figure **16.7**

Optic nerve, axial view, magnified.

Optic nerve (II)

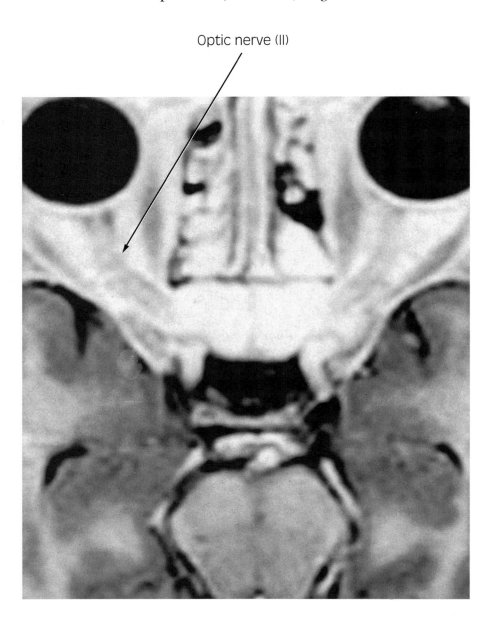

Figure **16.8**

Optic nerve, axial view, magnified.

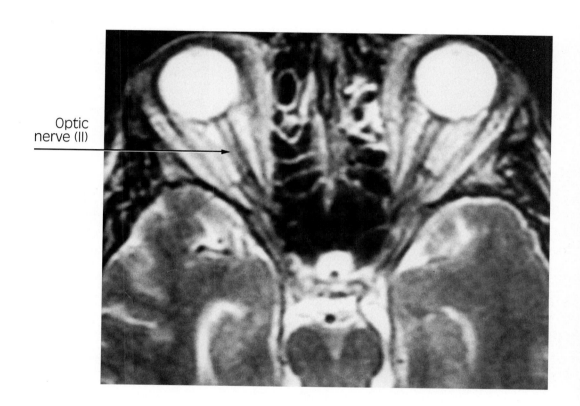

Optic
nerve (II)

Figure **16.9**

Optic nerve pathway, axial view.

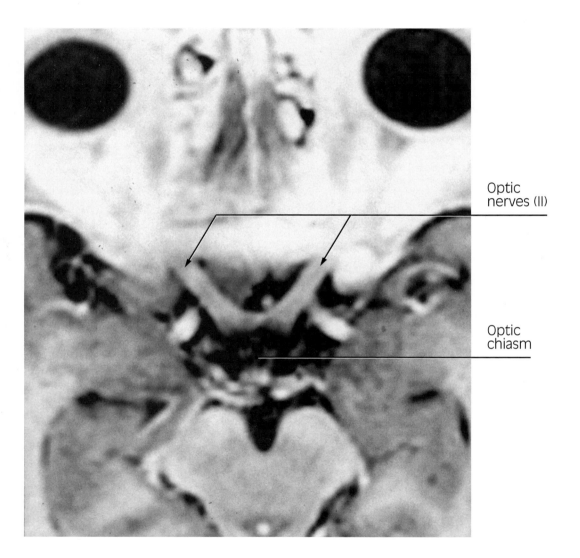

Optic
nerves (II)

Optic
chiasm

Figure **16.10**

Optic nerve pathway, axial view, magnified.

Optic tract

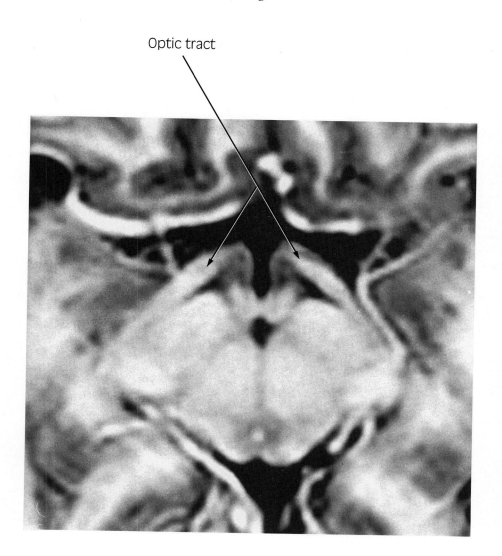

Figure **16.11**

Optic nerve pathway, sagittal view, magnified.

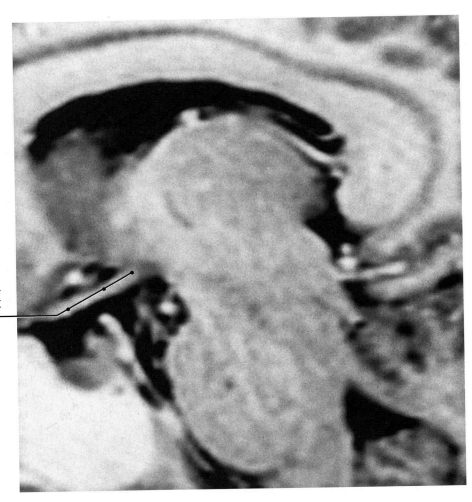

Optic nerve–
chiasm–tract

Figure **16.12**

Optic nerve pathway, sagittal view, magnified.

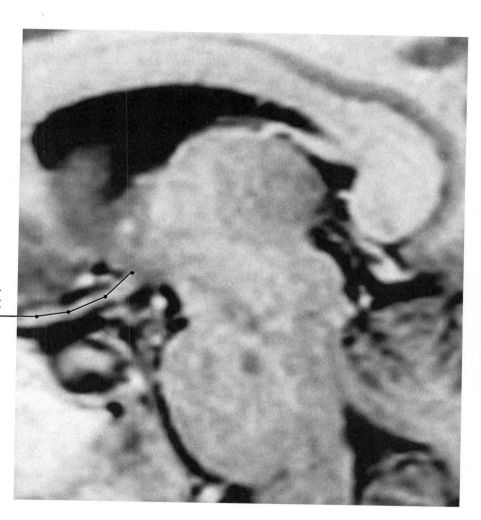

Optic nerve–
chiasm–tract

## From Midbrain

### Third Cranial Nerve: Oculomotor
(Figures **16.13** and **16.14**)

Demonstration:   Just posterior to the red nucleus and anterior to the superior aspect of the cerebral aqueduct

Supply:   Motor: Eye movement muscles and levator palpebrae

Parasympathetic: Smooth muscles of the eyeball

### Fourth Cranial Nerve: Trochlear
(Figure **16.15**)

Demonstration:   Just below the nucleus of cranial nerve III, and anterior to the aqueduct of Sylvius

Supply:   Motor: Superior oblique

Figure **16.13**

Oculomotor cranial nerve, sagittal view, magnified.

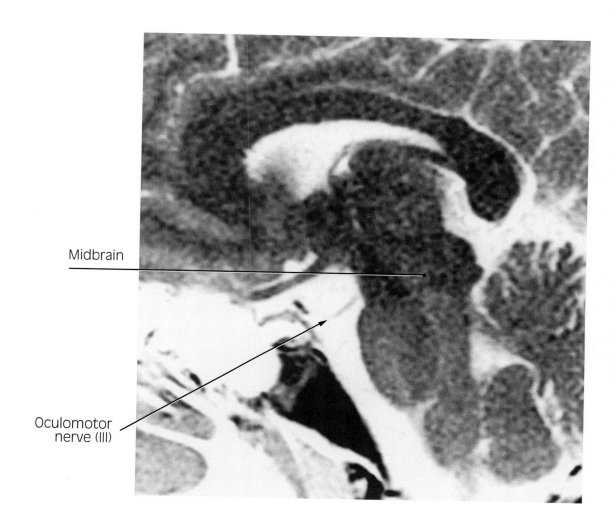

Midbrain

Oculomotor
nerve (III)

Figure **16.14**

Oculomotor and trochlear cranial nerves, sagittal view, magnified.

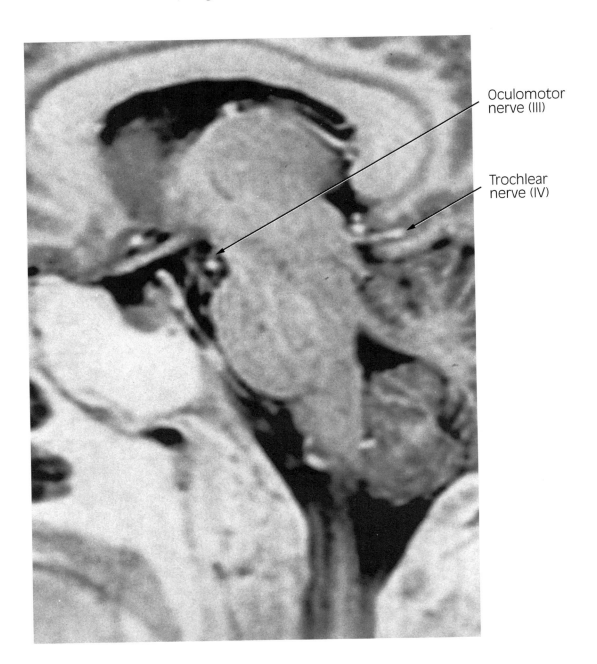

Oculomotor
nerve (III)

Trochlear
nerve (IV)

Figure **16.15**

Trochlear cranial nerve, sagittal view, magnified.

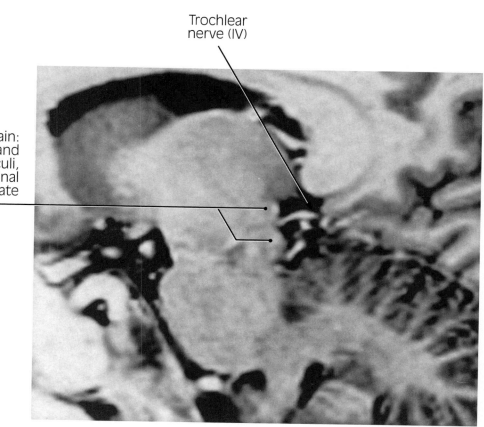

Trochlear
nerve (IV)

Midbrain:
superior and
inferior colliculi,
quadrigeminal
plate

## From Pons

### Fifth Cranial Nerve: Trigeminal
(Figure **16.16**)

Demonstration:   Lateral aspect of the pons and courses anteriorly in meckel's cave

Supply:   V1: Sensory: Forehead, eye, superior nasal cavities

V2: Sensory: Teeth, mucosa of superior mouth

V3: Sensory: Surface of jaw, lower teeth, mucosa of lower mouth, and anterior tongue

Motor: Muscles of mastication

Figure **16.16**

Trigeminal cranial nerve, axial view, magnified.

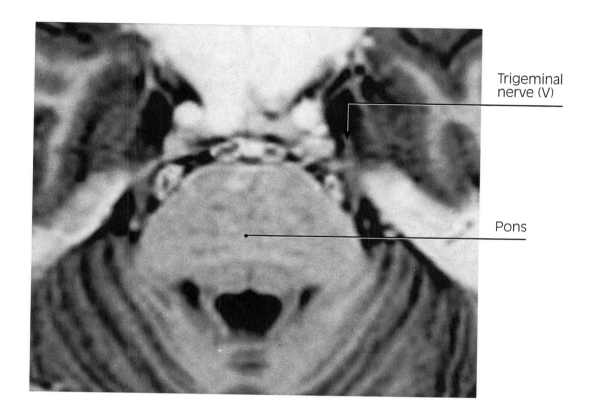

Trigeminal
nerve (V)

Pons

## Sixth Cranial Nerve: Abducent
(Figure **16.17**)

**Demonstration:**   In the middle of the pons, near the floor of the fourth ventricle

**Supply:**   Motor: Lateral rectus

Figure **16.17**

Abducent cranial nerve, axial view, magnified.

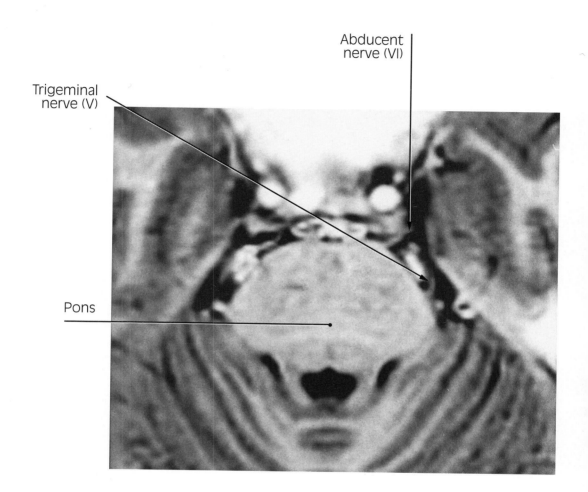

## Seventh Cranial Nerve: Facial
(Figures **16.18** and **16.19**)

Demonstration:  Anterolateral to the nucleus of the sixth cranial nerve

Supply:  Motor: Facial and cheek muscle, buccinator

## Eighth Cranial Nerve: Acoustic
(see Figures **16.18** and **16.19**)

Demonstration:  Superior aspect of the medulla along the base of the inferior cerebellar peduncle (vestibular nuclei more medial than the cochlear nuclei)

Supply:  Sensory: Vestibular and cochlear apparatus

Figure **16.18**

Facial and acoustic cranial nerves,
axial view, magnified.

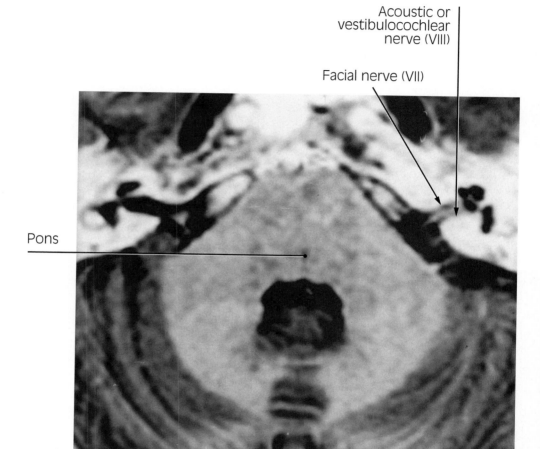

Acoustic or
vestibulocochlear
nerve (VIII)

Facial nerve (VII)

Pons

Figure **16.19a**

Cranial nerves, facial and acoustic nerves, axial view, magnified.

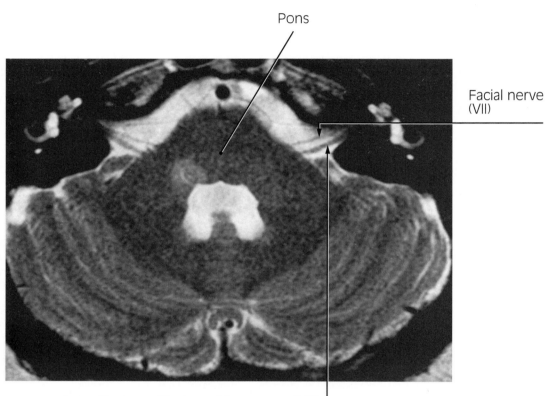

Pons

Facial nerve (VII)

Acoustic or vestibulocochlear nerve (VIII)

Figure **16.19b**

Facial and acoustic cranial nerves,
axial view, magnified.

Facial
nerve (VII)

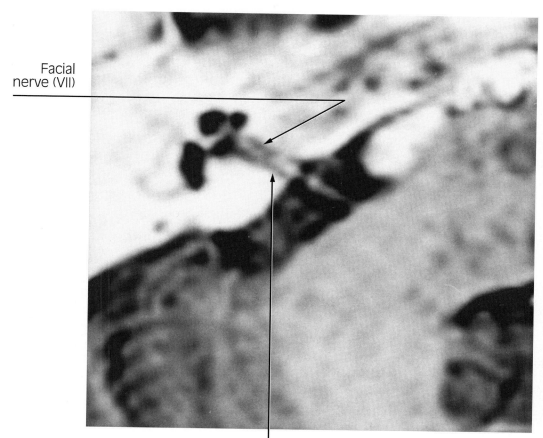

Acoustic or vestibulocochlear
nerve (VIII)

## From Medulla
(Figures **16.20** to **16.23**)

### Ninth Cranial Nerve: Glossopharyngeal

Demonstration:   Just posterior to the inferior olivary nucleus

Supply:   Sensory: Pharynx, posterior tongue

Motor: Superior pharyngeal muscles

### Tenth Cranial Nerve: Vagus

Demonstration:   Dorsal nucleus just anterior to the fourth ventricle in its inferior aspect

Supply:   Sensory: Thoracic and abdominal viscera

Motor: Larynx, middle and inferior pharyngeal muscles

Parasympathetic: Heart, lungs, and GI tract

### Eleventh Cranial Nerve: Spinal Accessory

Demonstration:   Lower medulla and upper cervical cord

Supply:   Motor: Sternomastoid and trapezius

### Twelfth Cranial Nerve: Hypoglossal
(Figure **16.24**)

Demonstration:   Along the paramedian area of the anterior wall of the fourth ventricle in the medulla

Supply:   Motor: Intrinsic muscles of tongue

Figure 16.20

Lower cranial nerves, axial view, magnified.

Lower
cranial nerve
complex

Medulla

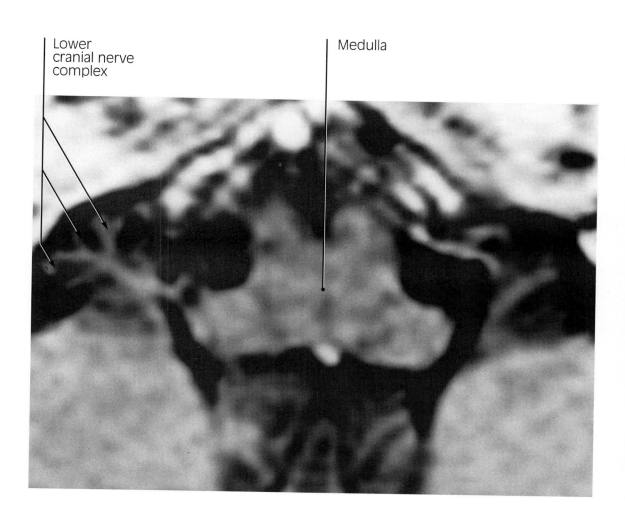

Figure **16.21**

Lower cranial nerves, axial view, magnified.

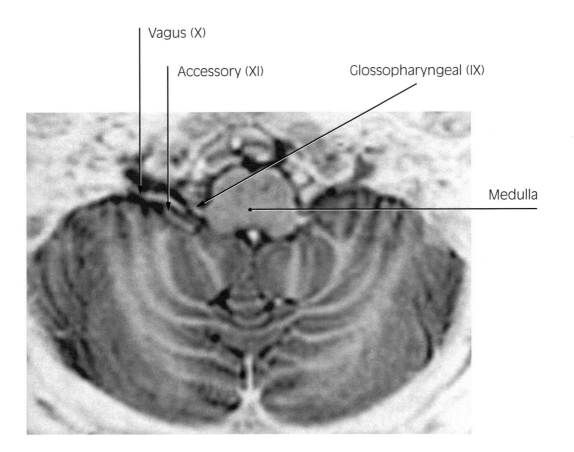

Vagus (X)

Accessory (XI)

Glossopharyngeal (IX)

Medulla

Figure **16.22**

Lower cranial nerves, axial view, magnified.

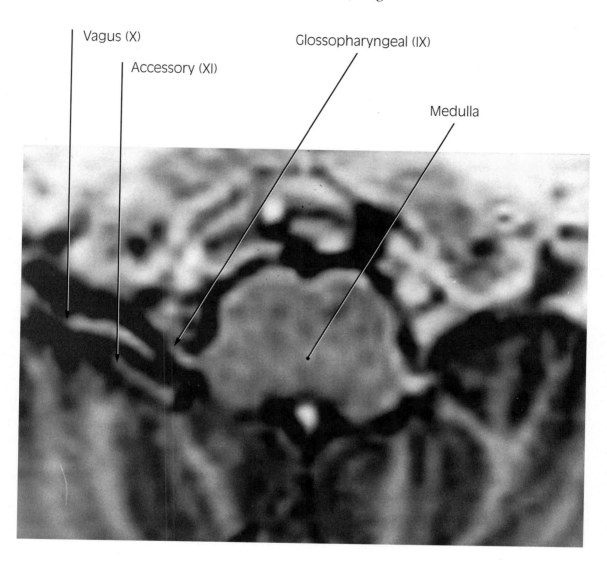

Vagus (X)

Accessory (XI)

Glossopharyngeal (IX)

Medulla

Figure **16.23**

Vagus cranial nerve, coronal view, magnified.

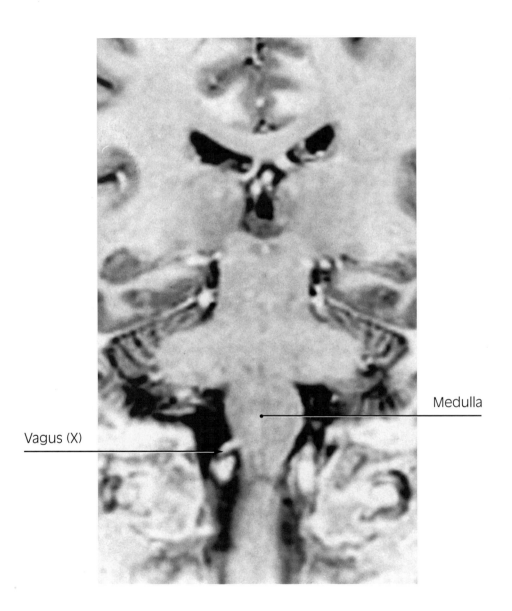

Medulla

Vagus (X)

Figure **16.24**

Hypoglossal cranial nerve, axial view.

Lower medulla

Hypoglossal
nerve (XI)

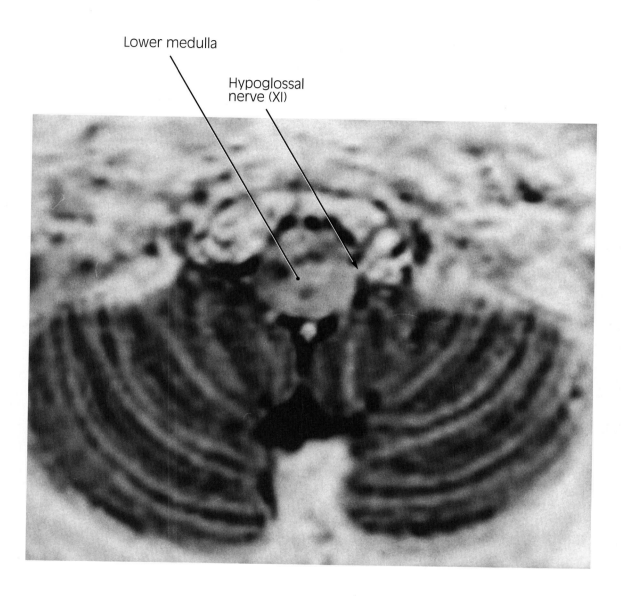

# CHAPTER 17

# Vascular Anatomy:
# Arterial System

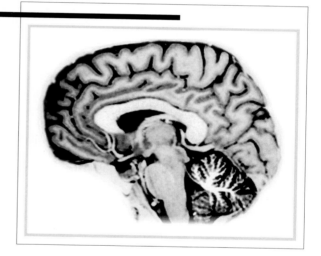

**Consists of two pairs of vessels and their branches:** Internal carotid arteries (ICAs)

Vertebral arteries

**Four ICA segments:** Cervical

Petrous

Cavernous

Intracranial/supraclinoid

**Cavernous + supraclinoid segments** ⟫ S-shaped loop or carotid siphon

**Cavernous segments:** Ascending: C5

Posterior genu: C4

Horizontal: C3

Anterior genu: C2

Intradural: C1

ICA enters the cranial fossa through the carotid canal and lies within the cavernous sinus.

# Cranial Arterial Supply

## Internal Carotid Artery Branches

| Branch | Supply |
|---|---|
| Ophthalmic | Central artery of retina |
| Posterior communicating (PCoA) | Optic chiasm and tract<br>Hypothalamus<br>Subthalamus<br>Anterior ventral thalamus |
| Anterior choroidal (AChA) | Temporal horn of choroid plexus<br>Hippocampus<br>Amygdala<br>Optic tract<br>Lateral geniculate body<br>Globus pallidus<br>Internal capsule, posterior limb<br>Optic radiation, proximal portion |

Anterior cerebral (ACA)

Frontal and parietal lobes, medial surface
Corpus callosum, medial surface
Optic chiasm
Caudate nucleus
Putamen
Internal capsule, anterior limb
Paracentral lobule, leg and foot areas

Anterior communicating (ACoA)

Connects the anterior cerebral arteries

Middle cerebral (MCA)

Cerebral hemisphere, lateral convexity
Insula
Motor and sensory cortex, trunk, arm, face
Insula
Motor and sensory cortex, trunk, arm, face
Speech areas, Broca's and Wernicke's
Caudate nucleus
Lentiform nuclei
Internal capsule, both limbs
Caudate nucleus
Lentiform nuclei
Internal capsule, both limbs

## Vertebral Arteries

| Branch | Supply |
| --- | --- |
| Anterior and posterior spinal | Spinal cord |
| Posterior inferior cerebellar (PICA) | Medulla, dorsolateral zone<br>Cerebellum, inferior surface<br>Fourth ventricle, choroid plexus<br>Vestibular nuclei, medial and inferior<br>Inferior cerebellar peduncles<br>Nucleus ambiguus<br>Glossopharyngeal and vagal intraaxial fibers<br>Spinothalamic tract<br>Spinal trigeminal tract |

## Basilar Artery

| Branch | Supply |
|---|---|
| Pontine | Corticospinal tracts<br>Abducent nerve intraaxial fibers |
| Labyrinthine | Cochlea and vestibular structures |
| Anterior inferior cerebellar (AICA) | Inferior cerebellar peduncles<br>Middle cerebellar peduncles<br>Spinothalamic tract<br>Spinal trigeminal nucleus and tract<br>Cochlear and vestibular nuclei<br>Facial and vestibular intraaxial fibers |
| Superior cerebellar | Superior cerebellar peduncles<br>Cerebellum, superior surface<br>Dentate nucleus<br>Pons, lateral and rostral portion<br>Spinothalamic tract |
| Posterior cerebral (PCA) | Midbrain<br>Thalamus, posterior half<br>Medial geniculate body<br>Lateral geniculate body<br>Occipital lobe<br>Visual cortex |
| Medial and lateral posterior choroidal (branch of the posterior cerebral) | Dorsal thalamus<br>Pineal gland<br>Lateral and third ventricle, choroid plexus |
| Penetrating arteries from circle of Willis | Hypothalamus<br>Subthalamus<br>Thalamus<br>Midbrain |

## Circle of Willis

The following form the arterial network of the circle of Willis. (Figures **17.1** to **17.6**)

- Anterior cerebral arteries, horizontal or A1 segments
- Anterior communicating arteries
- Internal carotid arteries
- Posterior communicating arteries
- Posterior cerebral arteries, horizontal or P1 segments
- Basilar artery (BA) tip

Figure **17.1**

MR arterial angiogram, lateral or sagittal,
segments of cavernous ICA.

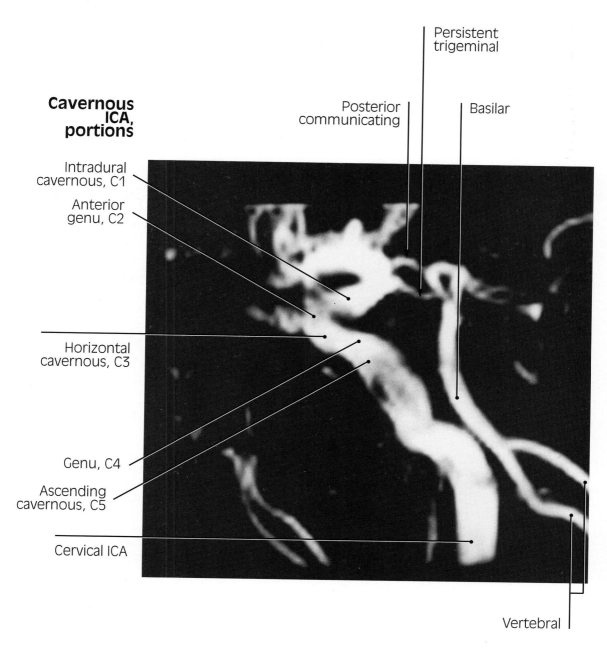

Persistent
trigeminal

Posterior
communicating

Basilar

**Cavernous
ICA,
portions**

Intradural
cavernous, C1

Anterior
genu, C2

Horizontal
cavernous, C3

Genu, C4

Ascending
cavernous, C5

Cervical ICA

Vertebral

## Anatomic Variations

| Artery | Important Variations |
| --- | --- |
| Circle of Willis | 75% with hypoplastic or absent segment(s) |
| ACoA | Hypoplasia<br>Duplication<br>Triplication |
| ACA | Infraoptic origin<br>Hypoplastic or absent A1 segment<br>Single ACA supplying both hemispheres<br>Duplication |
| ICA | Persistent trigeminal<br>Middle meningeal from ophthalmic artery |
| PCoA | Hypoplasia |
| PCA | Hypoplastic or absent P1 segment<br>Direct origin from ICA<br>Fetal origin |
| MCA | Nondivision of the main trunk<br>Partial duplication<br>Accessory MCA from ACA A1 segment<br>Duplication<br>Triplication<br>Quadrification |
| Basilar | Highly variable course |
| Vertebral | Hypoplasia<br>End in posterior inferior cerebellar<br>Duplication<br>Absence |

Figure **17.2**

MR arterial angiogram, sagittal oblique view.

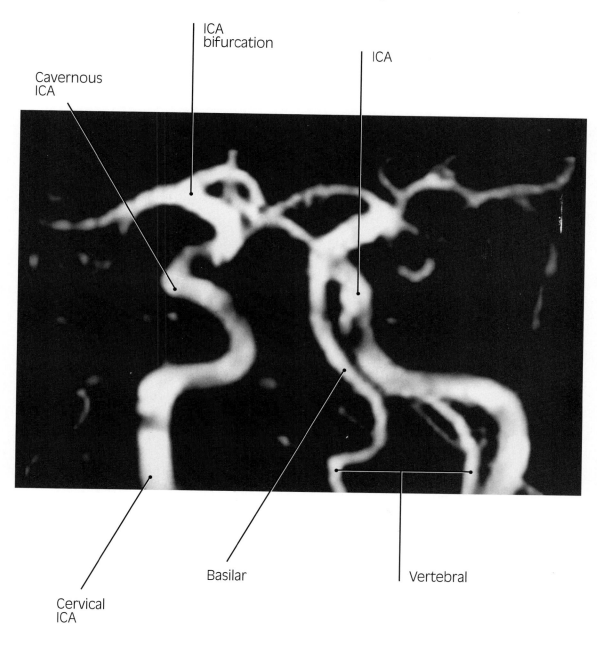

ICA
bifurcation

ICA

Cavernous
ICA

Basilar

Vertebral

Cervical
ICA

## Points to Remember

Normal cranial blood flow is 50 ml/100 g of brain tissue per minute.

The ACA supplies the anterior limb of the internal capsule via the medial striate artery of Hubner.

The MCA supplies the anterior and posterior limbs of the internal capsule via the lateral striate artery.

The vertebral arteries join to form the basilar artery at the junction between the medulla and the pons.

The posterior spinal artery is usually a branch of the posterior inferior cerebellar artery.

The labyrinthine artery is usually a branch of the anterior inferior cerebellar artery.

Bifurcation of the basilar artery forms the PCA.

### PRACTICAL POINTS

Thrombosis of one of the lenticulostriate branches of the MCA results in a lesion of the internal capsule and upper motor neuron type of paralysis.

Hemorrhage of Charcot's artery (one of the lenticulostriate branches also known as the artery of cerebral intraparenchymal hemorrhage) results in hemiplegia with a deep coma.

Thrombosis of Hubner's branch of the ACA causes contralateral upper monoplegia.

Thrombosis of the terminal cortical branch of the ACA causes contralateral lower monoplegia.

Wallenberg's lateral medullary syndrome is due to thrombosis of the posterior inferior cerebellar artery.

Figure **17.3**

MR arterial angiogram, sagittal oblique view.

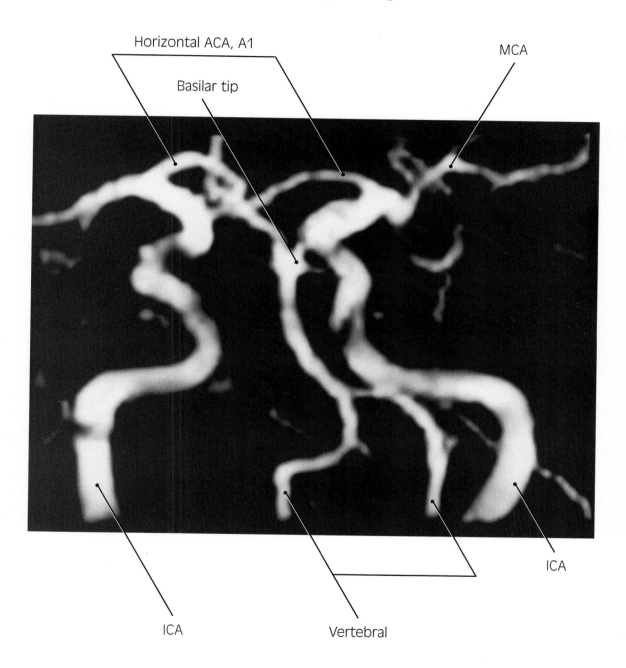

Horizontal ACA, A1

Basilar tip

MCA

ICA

ICA

Vertebral

## Incidence of Aneurysms

| Arteries | Aneurysm (%) |
|---|---|
| ACoA | 30–35 |
| ICA | 30–35 |
| PCoA | 30–35 |
| MCA bifurcation | 20 |
| Basilar | 5 |
| Superior and inferior cerebellar | 5 |
| AChA | 1–3 |
| Pericallosal | 1–3 |

Figure **17.4**

MR arterial angiogram.

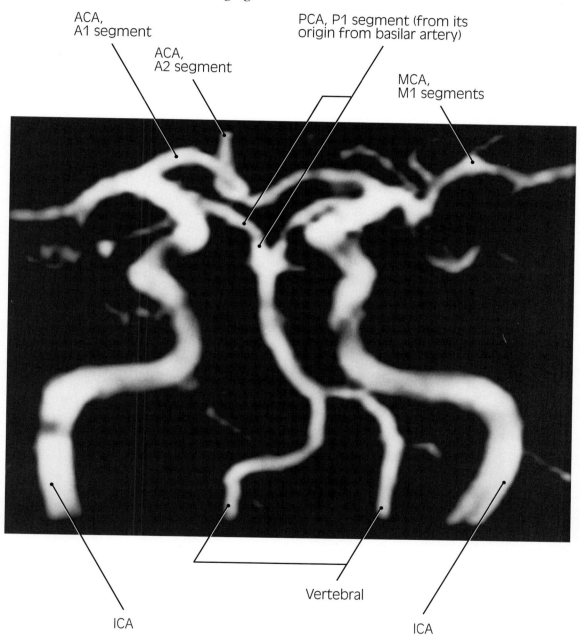

ACA,
A1 segment

ACA,
A2 segment

PCA, P1 segment (from its
origin from basilar artery)

MCA,
M1 segments

ICA

Vertebral

ICA

Figure **17.5**

## MR arterial angiogram, circle of Willis.

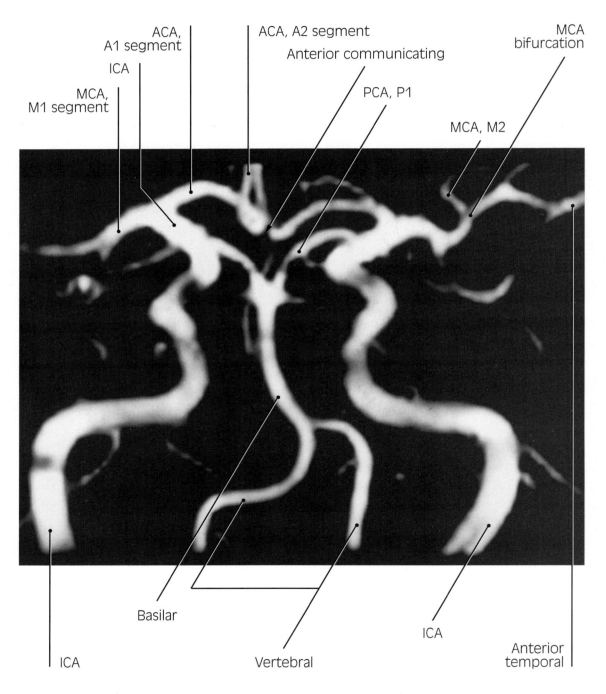

ACA,
A1 segment

ICA

MCA,
M1 segment

ACA, A2 segment

Anterior communicating

PCA, P1

MCA
bifurcation

MCA, M2

Basilar

Vertebral

ICA

ICA

Anterior
temporal

Figure **17.6**

MR arterial angiogram, circle of Willis.

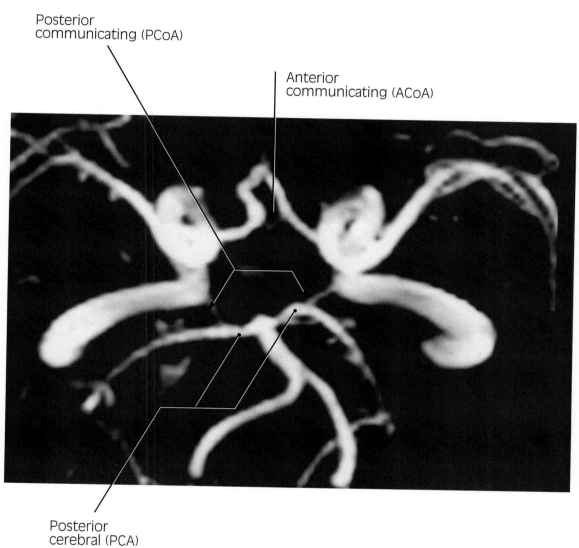

Posterior
communicating (PCoA)

Anterior
communicating (ACoA)

Posterior
cerebral (PCA)

CHAPTER *18*

# Vascular Anatomy: Venous System

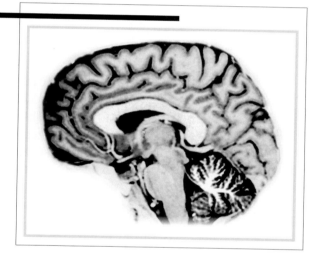

Cerebral veins that empty into the dural sinuses drain blood from the brain. They are drained mostly by the internal jugular veins (IJVs).

## Dural Sinuses

### Superior Sagittal Sinus (SSS)

Appearance:   Triangular in cross-section

Location:   In the attached border of the falx cerebri

Origin:   At the foramen cecum

Course:   Runs backward toward the internal occipital protuberance (IOP)

Termination:   At the IOP, it joins with the straight sinus (SS) and lateral sinuses (LSs) and forms the torcular Herophili

Drainage:   Major cerebral cortex + scalp

**N O T E**   The anterior part of the SSS is narrow and sometimes absent, or is replaced by two superior cerebral veins that join behind the coronal suture. This is why the anterior part of the sinus is often poorly visualized, and isolated lack of filling is not sufficient to suggest thrombosis.

### Inferior Sagittal Sinus (ISS)

Location:   Inferior free margins of falx

Course:   Posterior

Meets:   Internal cerebral vein (ICV)

### Lateral Sinuses (LSs)

Course:   Extend from the torcular Herophili to jugular bulbs

Parts:   Transverse (TS): In the attached border of the tentorium

Sigmoid: On the inner aspect of the mastoid process

Drainage:   Posterior cerebral cortex + cerebellum + brain stem + middle ears

**N O T E**   The right transverse sinus is frequently larger than the left.

## Torcular Herophili

Formation:   Confluences of SSS and SS

Branches:   Bifurcates into two TS (part of LS)

## Cavernous Sinuses (CSs)

Location:   On either side of the sella turcica, superolaterally to the sphenoid air sinuses

Contents:   Consist of trabeculated cavities formed by separation of the layers of the dura

Termination:   Empty into both the superior and inferior petrosal sinuses

Drainage:   Orbits + anterior basal brain

## Straight Sinus (SS)

Formation:   Union of the inferior sagittal sinus and the great vein of Galen

Appearance:   Triangular

Location:   Between the falx cerebri and the tentorium cerebelli

Termination:   Joins the torcular at the IOP

## Cerebral Veins

### Superficial Cerebral or Cortical Veins

Frontal, parietal, and occipital → SSS

Middle cerebral veins (MCVs) → CS

SSS → vein of Trolard → MCV → vein of Labbé → LS

### Deep Cerebral Veins

Thalamostriate + septal → ICV

ICV + basal vein of Rosenthal → vein of Galen → SS

# MR Venous (MRV) Angiography

## Two-Dimensional Time of Flight Venous Angiogram

For the complete assessment of the superficial and deep venous system and the dural sinuses, it is important to obtain the following reconstructive images.
(Figures **18.1** to **18.13**)

| Reconstruction | Sinuses |
| --- | --- |
| Axial | Lateral sinuses |
| Coronal | Superior sagittal sinus <br> Lateral sinuses <br> Cavernous sinus <br> Cortical veins |
| Sagittal | Posterior SSS <br> Deep venous system <br> Vein of Galen <br> Lateral sinus <br> Straight sinus <br> Cortical veins |

## FUNCTIONAL CONSIDERATIONS

Cortical veins or sinus thrombosis: Dehydration
Mastoiditis
Postpartum
Polycythemia

Meningeal and sinus invasions by tumors such as meningiomas

Vascular malformations

Low position of the torcular Herophili or TS: Chiari II
malformation

Figure **18.1**

MR venous angiogram, axial view.

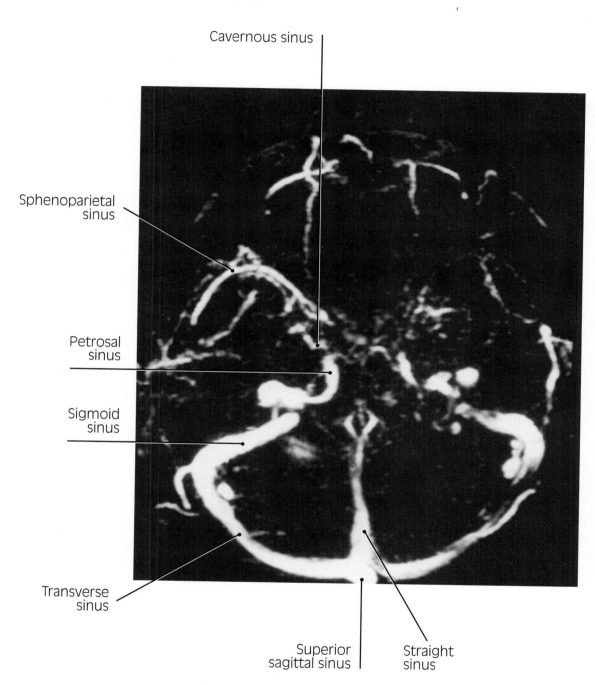

Cavernous sinus

Sphenoparietal sinus

Petrosal sinus

Sigmoid sinus

Transverse sinus

Superior sagittal sinus

Straight sinus

## Blood-Brain Barriers

The nervous system is isolated from the blood by a barrier system that provides a stable environment for neurologic functions.

The components of blood-brain barriers (BBB) are as follows:

Choroid plexus of the ventricle

Pineal gland

Pituitary gland

Median eminence

Subcommissural organs

Subforniceal organs

Area postrema

Organum vasculosum of the lamina terminalis

Metabolic water is the only component of CSF that does not cross the blood-brain barriers.

**Breakdowns of BBB:**   Trauma

Spontaneous hemorrhage

Infection (meningitis)

Tumors

Hypercapnic conditions

Hypertensive encephalopathy

**Functions of BBB:**   Regulate entry of glucose

Control sodium influx in CSF

Control potassium efflux in blood

Prevent toxic effects of metabolites

Figure **18.2**

MR venous angiogram, sagittal view.

Superior sagittal
sinus (SSS)

Straight
sinus

SSS

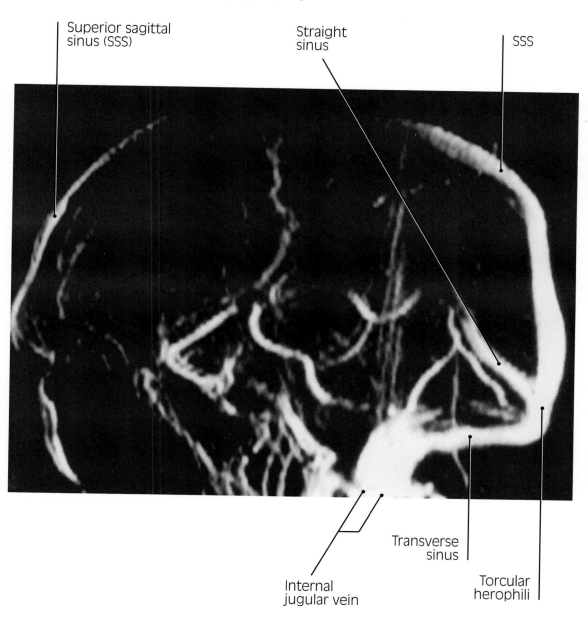

Internal
jugular vein

Transverse
sinus

Torcular
herophili

Figure **18.3**

MR venous angiogram, sagittal view.

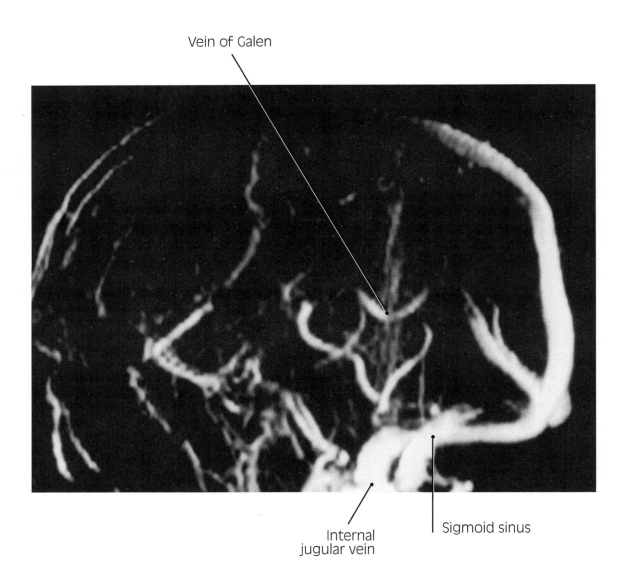

Vein of Galen

Internal
jugular vein

Sigmoid sinus

Figure **18.4**

MR venous anigogram, sagittal view.

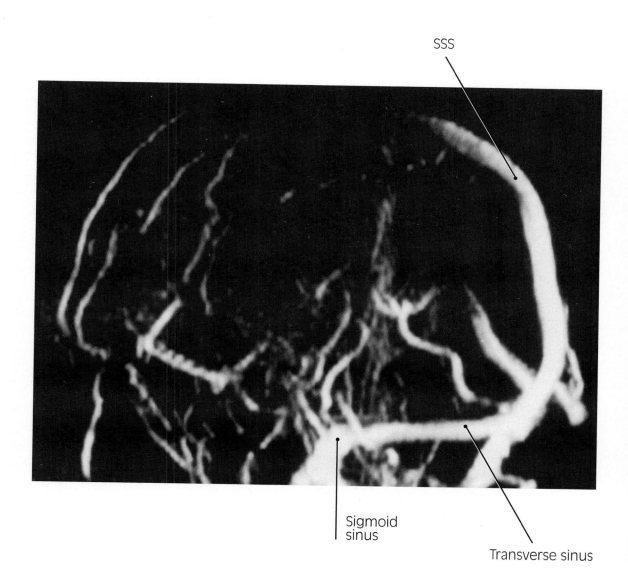

SSS

Sigmoid
sinus

Transverse sinus

Figure **18.5**

MR venous angiogram, sagittal view.

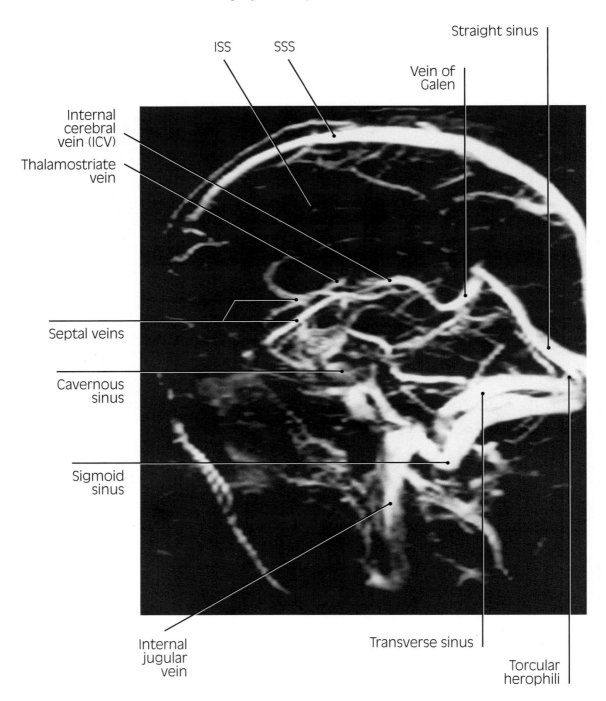

Figure **18.6**

MR venous angiogram, sagittal view.

Septal
vein

Thalamostriate
vein

Internal
cerebral
vein

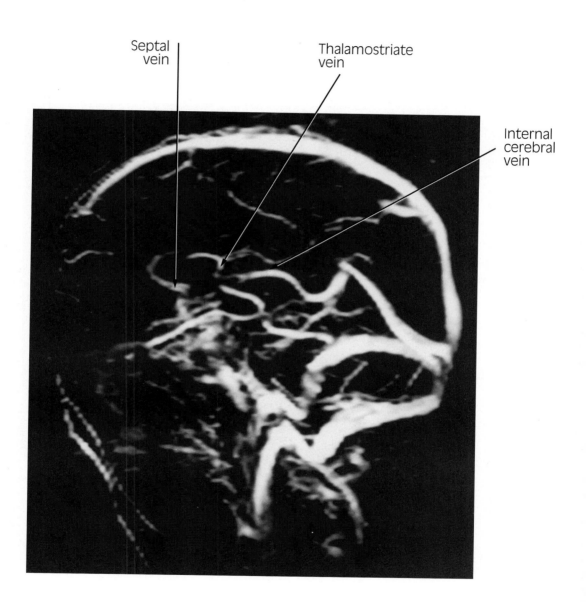

Figure **18.7**

MR venous angiogram, sagittal format with 90-degree rotation.

Sigmoid
sinus

Transverse
sinus

SSS

SSS

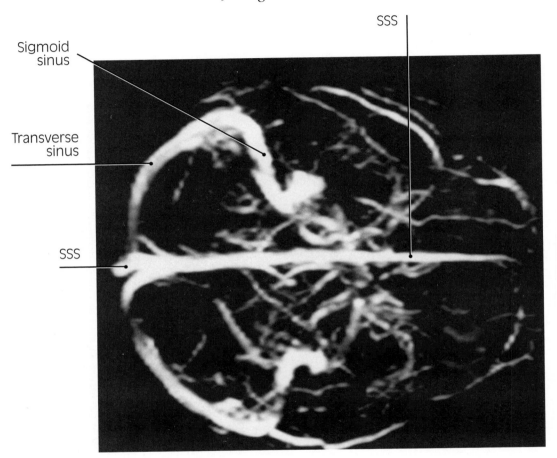

Figure **18.8**

MR venous angiogram, sagittal view.

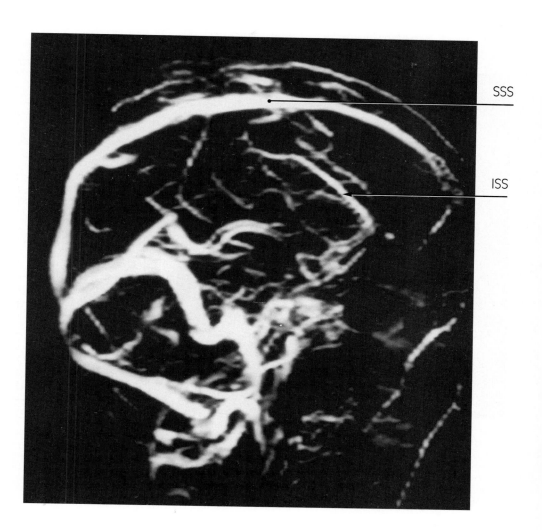

SSS

ISS

Figure **18.9**

MR venous angiogram, sagittal oblique view.

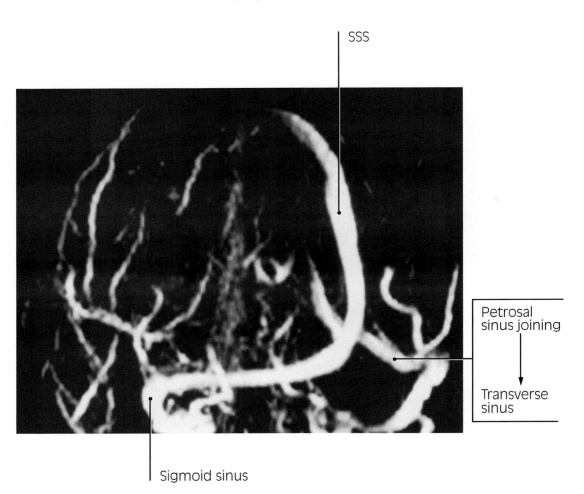

SSS

Petrosal
sinus joining

Transverse
sinus

Sigmoid sinus

Figure **18.10**

MR venous angiogram, coronal view.

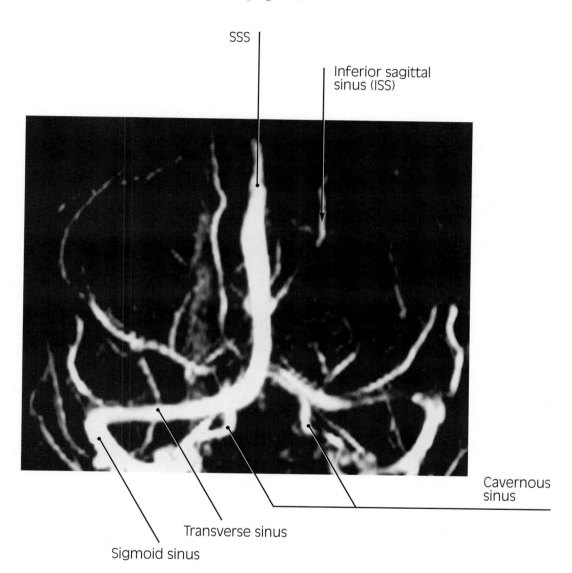

SSS

Inferior sagittal
sinus (ISS)

Cavernous
sinus

Transverse sinus

Sigmoid sinus

Figure **18.11**

MR venous angiogram, coronal format with 20-degree rotation.

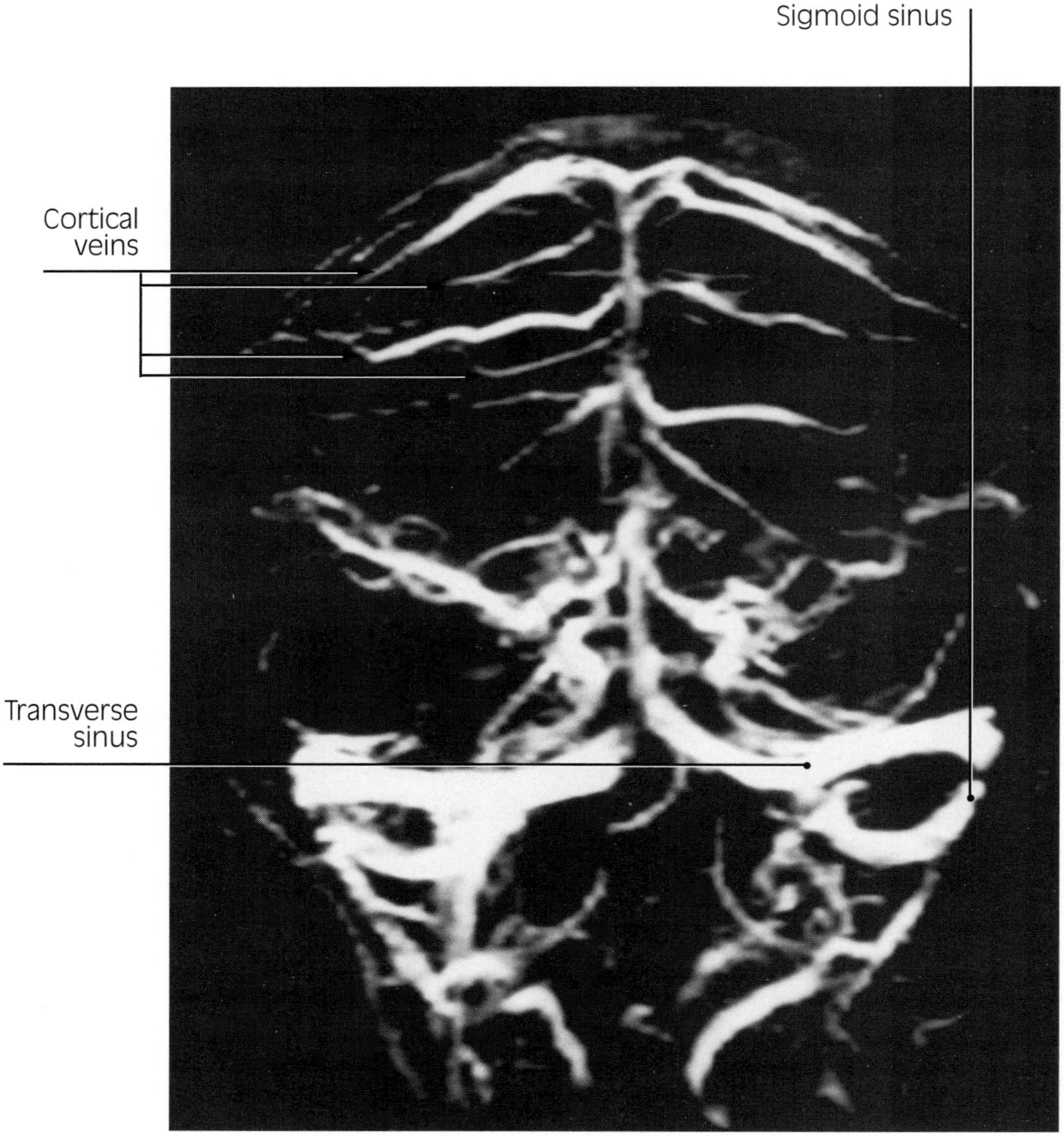

Figure **18.12**

MR venous angiogram, coronal view.

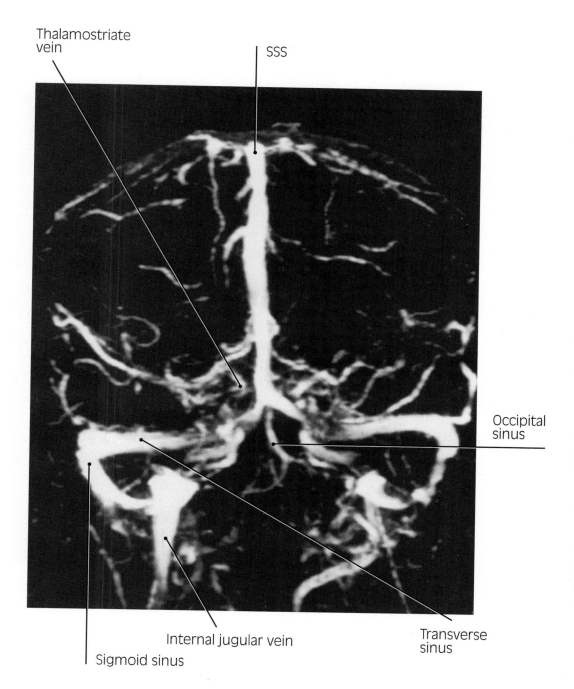

Thalamostriate vein

SSS

Occipital sinus

Internal jugular vein

Sigmoid sinus

Transverse sinus

Figure **18.13**

MR venous angiogram, coronal format with
90-degree rotation.

Spheno-
parietal
sinus

Cavernous
sinus

Sigmoid
sinus

Transverse
sinus

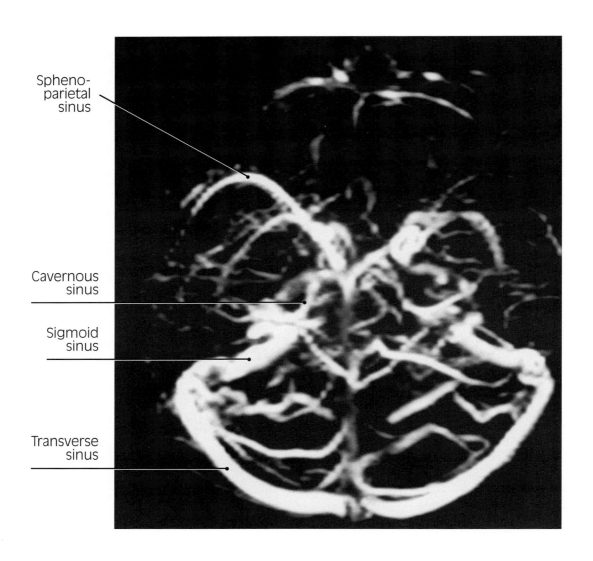

CHAPTER *19*

# Normal Anatomic Variations

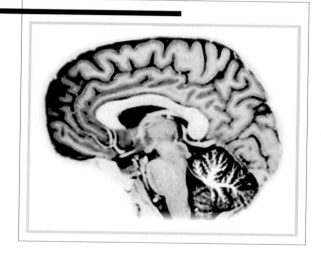

The advent of MRI, with its exquisite anatomic detail, high sensitivity, and multiplanar capability, has revolutionized imaging of the brain and spinal cord. MRI has superseded computed tomography (CT) as the best method of examination. However, there is more detail and information on any one standard MRI sequence than on CT, and therefore the task of reviewing MRI head scans can be daunting to the new radiologist. The following describes the normal anatomic variants encountered during routine MRI of the brain on a daily basis.

## Skull Vault

### Dural Calcification or Ossification
(Figures **19.1** to **19.3**)

Dural calcification or ossification (*see arrow on figures*) is a frequent finding in cranial CT imaging of the adult population, especially in the elderly, and can be misdiagnosed as meningioma or lipoma. Fatty marrow in the ossification is of high signal intensity on T1-weighted images and of low signal intensity on T2-weighted images.

Figure **19.1**

Skull vault, dural calcification or ossification (*arrow*), sagittal T1-weighted image.

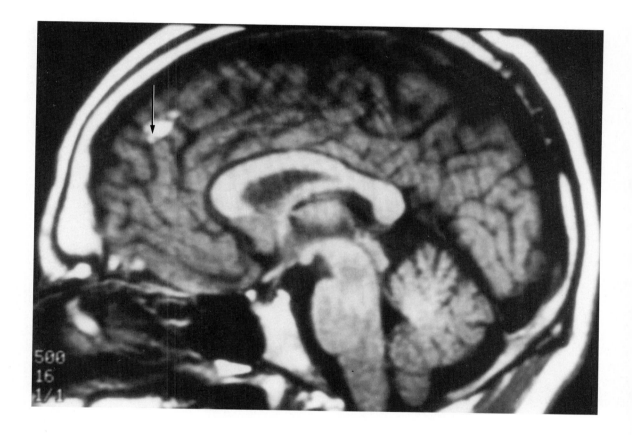

*Used with permission from Patel VH, Friedman L: Normal variations in MR imaging of the brain.* Seminars in Ultrasound, CT, and MRI *1995;16:175–185.*

Figure **19.2**

Skull vault, dural calcification or ossification (*arrow*), sagittal T1-weighted image.

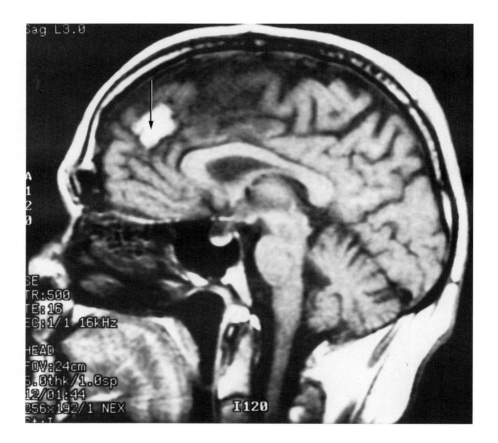

*Used with permission from Patel VH, Friedman L: Normal variations in MR imaging of the brain.* Seminars in Ultrasound, CT, and MRI *1995;16:175–185.*

Figure **19.3**

Skull vault, dural calcification or ossification (*arrow*),
axial T2-weighted image.

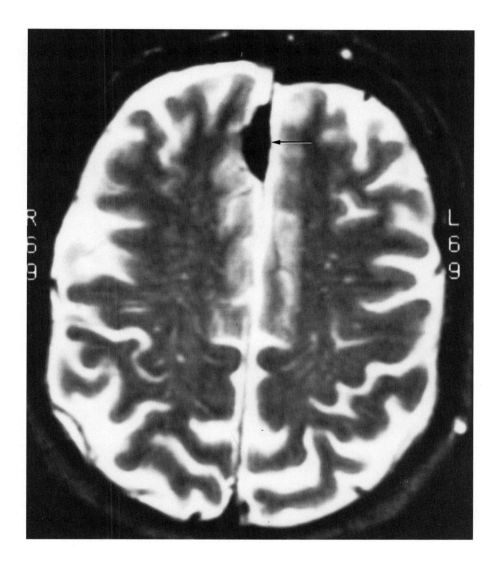

*Used with permission from Patel VH, Friedman L: Normal variations in MR imaging of the brain.* Seminars in
Ultrasound, CT, and MRI *1995;16:175–185.*

## Pacchionian Granulations
(Figure **19.4**)

Pacchionian granulations (*arrows*), when large, may simulate calvarial metastases. A size less than 2 to 3 cm, a parasagittal location, and a sessile configuration in the sagittal or coronal plane suggest their true entity. In addition, continuity to a dural sinus, sharp margins, and a grapelike or clustered appearance assist in the distinction from a pathologic process.

Figure **19.4**

Skull vault, pacchionian granulations (*arrows*),
coronal image.

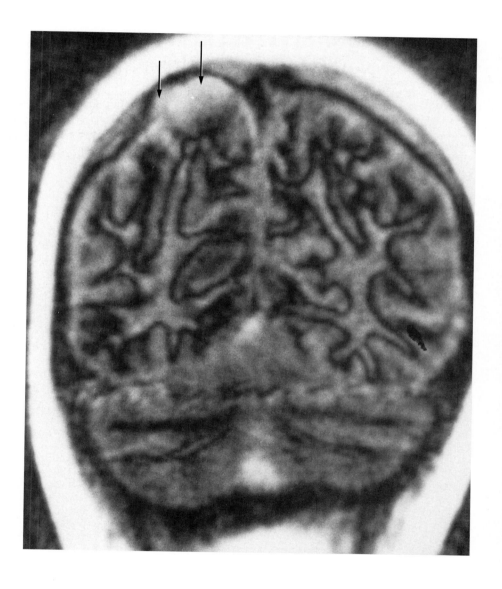

*Used with permission from Patel VH, Friedman L: Normal variations in MR imaging of the brain.*
Seminars in Ultrasound, CT, and MRI *1995;16:175–185.*

# Cerebral Cortex

## Gyrus Rectus
(Figure **19.5**)

On slightly offset midline sagittal T1-weighted images, hypointensity of the gray matter of the gyrus rectus (*arrows*) may simulate a midline lesion in the frontal lobe. Careful assessment of the location of the signal and correlation with T2-weighted images will distinguish it from a genuine lesion.

## Cerebral Cortex Pseudolesions
(Figures **19.6** and **19.7**)

Partial volume averaging of the cortices can result in apparent lesions. Important to note is that the "apparent" focus maintains the same signal characteristics (*arrows*) as the adjacent cortex. A true lesion appears much brighter on T2-weighted images.

Figure **19.5**

Cerebral cortex, gyrus rectus (*arrows*), sagittal T1-weighted image.

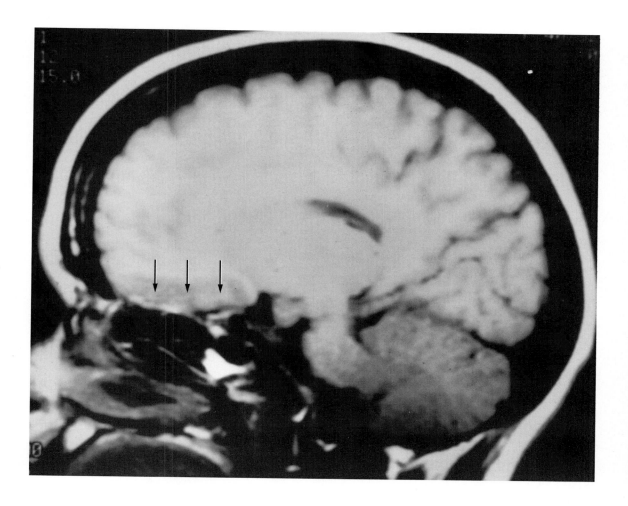

*Used with permission from Patel VH, Friedman L: Normal variations in MR imaging of the brain.*
Seminars in Ultrasound, CT, and MRI *1995;16:175–185.*

Figure **19.6**

Cerebral cortex, pseudolesions (*arrows*),
axial proton density image.

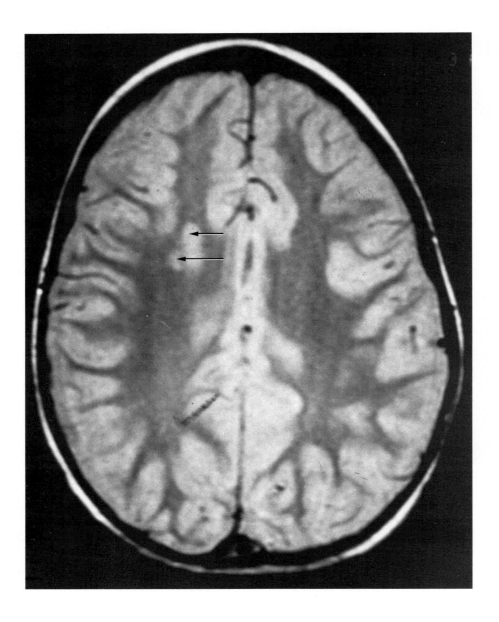

*Used with permission from Patel VH, Friedman L: Normal variations in MR imaging of the brain.* Seminars in Ultrasound, CT, and MRI *1995;16:175–185.*

Figure **19.7**

Cerebral cortex, pseudolesions (*arrows*),
axial T2-weighted image.

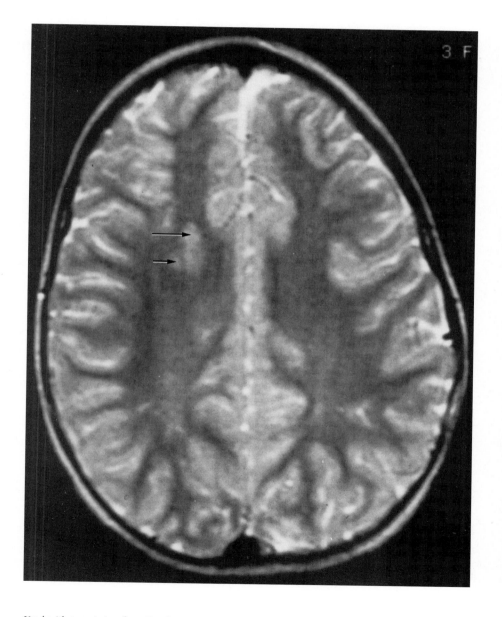

*Used with permission from Patel VH, Friedman L: Normal variations in MR imaging of the brain.*
Seminars in Ultrasound, CT, and MRI *1995;16:175–185.*

# White Matter Tracts

## Parietopontine Tract
(Figures **19.8** to **19.11**)

*Location*:   Medial to the distal putamen near the junction of the posterior limb and the retrolenticular portion of the internal capsule at the level of the velum interpositum.

*Appearance*:   The parietopontine tract (*arrows*) appears as a well-defined oval or round increased signal intensity relative to the rest of the internal capsule on axial T2-weighted images.

Figure **19.8**

White matter parietopontine tracts (*arrows*),
axial T2-weighted image.

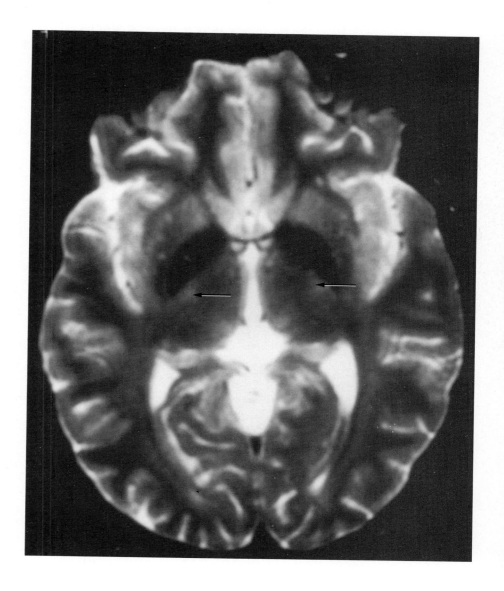

*Used with permission from Patel VH, Friedman L: Normal variations in MR imaging of the brain.*
Seminars in Ultrasound, CT, and MRI *1995;16:175–185.*

> **N O T E** This signal pattern results from less heavy myelination and is seen in nearly 50 percent of the adult population. It is iso- to hypointense on proton density images and hypointense on T1-weighted images.

## KEY FEATURE

The parietopontine tract is bilateral and mostly symmetrical, with definitely no mass effect or enhancement following gadolinium, and therefore one should not mistake it for an abnormal area of myelination.

Figure **19.9**

White matter parietopontine tracts (*arrows*),
axial T2-weighted image.

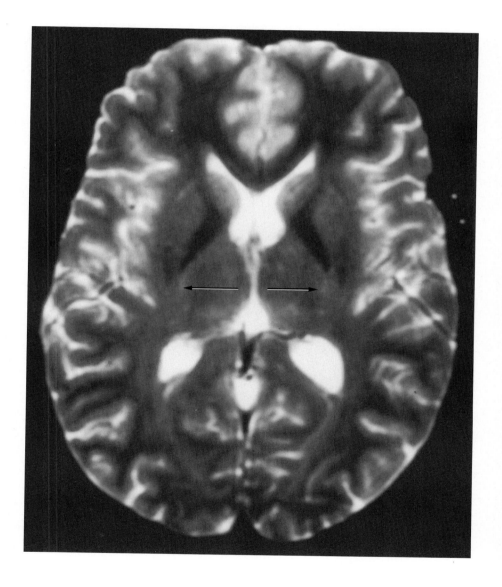

*Used with permission from Patel VH, Friedman L: Normal variations in MR imaging of the brain.*
Seminars in Ultrasound, CT, and MRI *1995;16:175–185.*

Figure **19.10**

White matter parietopontine tracts (*arrows*), axial FMPIR image with inverse video setting.

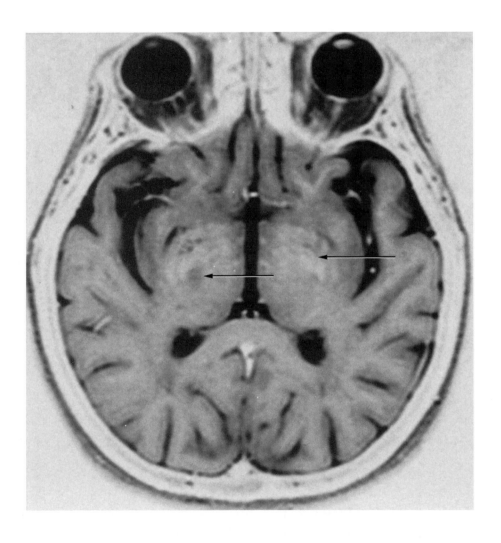

*Used with permission from Patel VH, Friedman L: Normal variations in MR imaging of the brain.* Seminars in Ultrasound, CT, and MRI *1995;16:175–185.*

Figure **19.11**

White matter parietopontine tracts (*arrows*),
axial T2-weighted image.

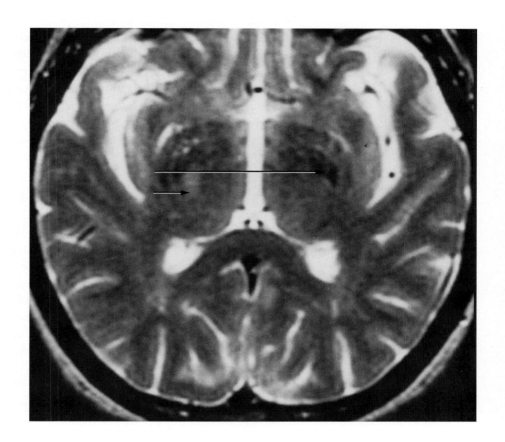

*Used with permission from Patel VH, Friedman L: Normal variations in MR imaging of the brain.*
Seminars in Ultrasound, CT, and MRI *1995;16:175–185.*

## Ependymitis Granularis
(Figure **19.12**)

*Location*:    Anterior and lateral to the frontal horns.

*Appearance*:    We see the ependymitis granularis (*arrows*) as high-signal-intensity foci on axial T2-weighted images.

---

**N O T E**    The high-signal-intensity appearance of ependymitis granularis is caused by (a) a decrease in myelination content, (b) a focal breakdown of the ependymal lining and gliosis, and (c) an increase in the periependymal extracellular fluid. We see it as an isointense to low-signal-intensity structure on proton density images and of low signal intensity on T1-weighted images.

---

**KEY FEATURES**

Ependymitis granularis is usually bilateral, essentially symmetrical, and commonly seen beside the frontal horns. In the appropriate age group and gender, one can differentiate these lesions from the lesions of multiple sclerosis on the basis of the following: (a) ependymitis granularis lesions are one on each side and usually less than 5 mm in size; (b) they are away from the callososeptal interface; (c) there is no further extension in the perivenular deep white matter; (d) there is a nonbeveled appearance on T1-weighted and proton density images; (e) there is no mass effect or enhancement following gadolinium; and (f) there is a negative history and noncontributing clinical presentation.

Figure **19.12**

White matter tracts, ependymitis granularis
(*arrows*), axial T2-weighted image.

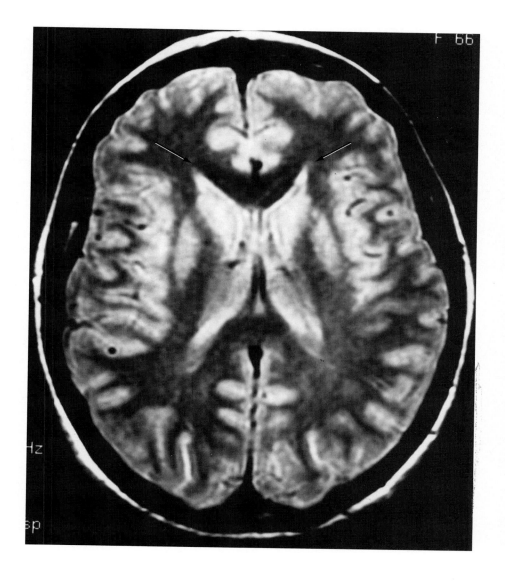

*Used with permission from Patel VH, Friedman L: Normal variations in MR imaging of the brain.*
Seminars in Ultrasound, CT, and MRI *1995;16:175–185.*

Figure **19.13**

White matter tracts, corpus callosum, sagittal T1-weighted image.

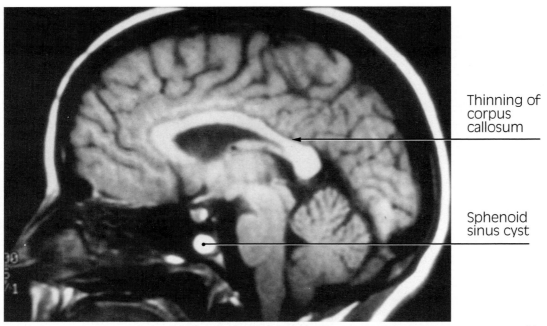

Thinning of corpus callosum

Sphenoid sinus cyst

*Used with permission from Patel VH, Friedman L: Normal variations in MR imaging of the brain.* Seminars in Ultrasound, CT, and MRI *1995;16:175–185.*

**Corpus Callosum**

**Thinning of the Corpus Callosum**

(Figures **19.13** and **19.14**)

*Location*:    Body of the corpus callosum.

*Appearance*:    We best visualize the corpus callosum on sagittal T1- and T2-weighted images. It exhibits high signal on T2-weighted images and low signal on T1-weighted images.

Figure **19.14**

White matter tracts, corpus callosum,
sagittal T1-weighted image.

Thinning
of corpus
callosum

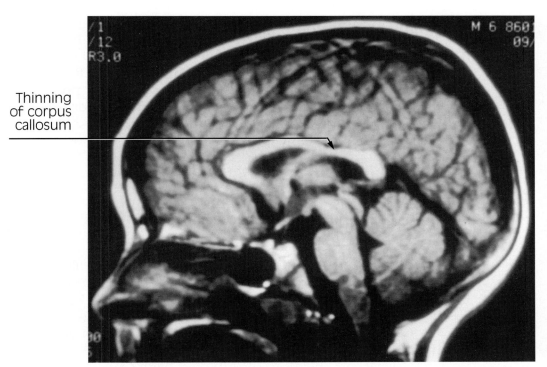

*Used with permission from Patel VH, Friedman L: Normal variations in MR imaging of the brain.*
Seminars in Ultrasound, CT, and MRI *1995;16:175–185.*

**NOTE** With partial callosal agenesis the rostrum and splenium are
absent or hypoplastic and the genu and body are present to
various degrees. However, diffuse or localized thinning of the
body of the corpus callosum can occur as a normal variation.
This is best visualized on sagittal T1- and T2-weighted images.
Note the high-signal-intensity cyst in the sphenoid sinus in
Figure 19.13.

### Corpus Callosum Lipoma
(Figure **19.15**)

*Location*:    In the posterior portion of the corpus callosum.

*Appearance*:    Because of its fat content, the lipoma is typically high signal intensity on T1-weighted images and low signal intensity on T2-weighted images.

> **N O T E**    Thirty percent of all intracranial lipomas occur in the callosal area. Anteriorly situated tubulonodular types of corpus callosal lipomas are frequently associated with forebrain and rostral callosal anomalies. Although posteriorly present, curvilinear lipomas are generally seen with a normal or nearly normal corpus callosum, and therefore are considered a common incidental finding.

## Ventricles

### Lateral Ventricle Pseudolesions
(Figures **19.16** and **19.17**)

Asymmetry of the lateral ventricles due to a slight tilt of the head can result in an apparent high-signal lesion (*arrow*, Figure 19.16) in the region of the body of the corpus callosum on T2-weighted axial images. This is due to a partial volume effect through the superior aspect of the lateral ventricle. A corresponding normal proton density image (Figure 19.17) confirms that the apparent abnormal signal corresponds to cerebrospinal fluid (CSF) in the lateral ventricle and not a demyelinating plaque.

### Lateral Ventricle Temporal Horn Pseudolesions
(Figures **19.18** and **19.19**)

As with the lateral ventricles, asymmetry of the temporal horn of the lateral ventricle can mimic a lesion in the medial aspect of the temporal lobe. Reviewing consecutive scans and proton density images will help exclude pathology.

Figure **19.15**

White matter tracts, corpus callosum,
sagittal T1-weighted image.

Lipoma of
corpus callosum,
splenium

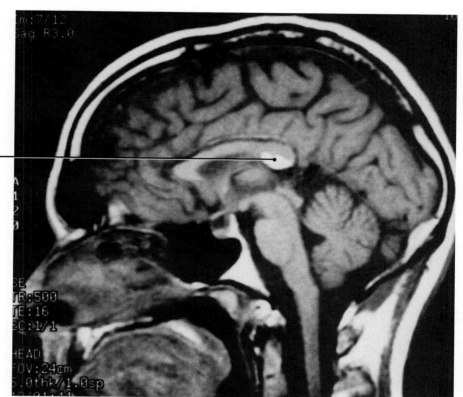

*Used with permission from Patel VH, Friedman L: Normal variations in MR imaging of the
brain.* Seminars in Ultrasound, CT, and MRI *1995;16:175–185.*

Figure **19.16**

Lateral ventricle, pseudolesions (*arrow*),
axial T2-weighted image.

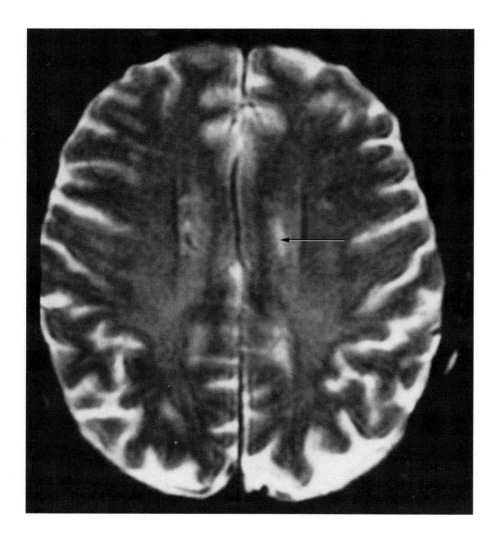

*Used with permission from Patel VH, Friedman L: Normal variations in MR imaging of the brain.* Seminars in Ultrasound, CT, and MRI *1995;16:175–185.*

Figure **19.17**

Lateral ventricle pseudolesions (*arrows*),
axial proton density image.

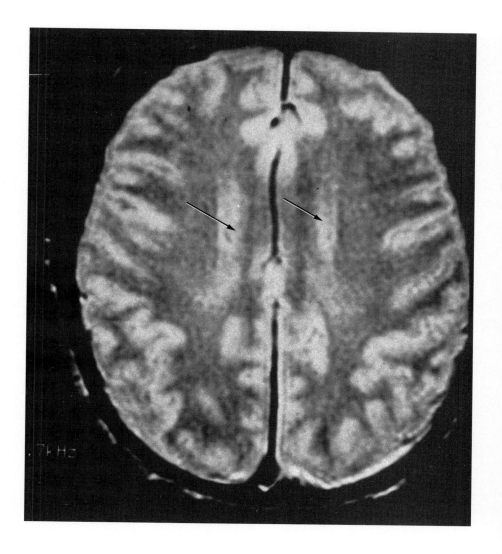

*Used with permission from Patel VH, Friedman L: Normal variations in MR imaging of the brain.*
Seminars in Ultrasound, CT, and MRI *1995;16:175–185.*

Figure **19.18**

Lateral ventricles, temporal horn (*arrow*, asymmetric appearance), axial T2-weighted image.

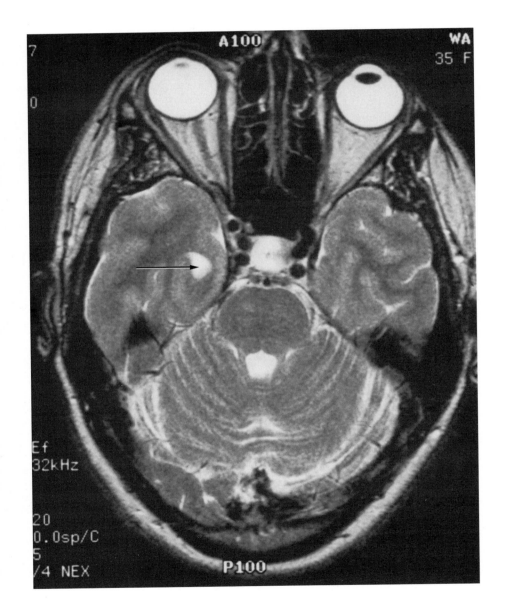

*Used with permission from Patel VH, Friedman L: Normal variations in MR imaging of the brain.* Seminars in Ultrasound, CT, and MRI *1995;16:175–185.*

Figure **19.19**

Lateral ventricles, temporal horns (*arrows*),
axial T2-weighted image.

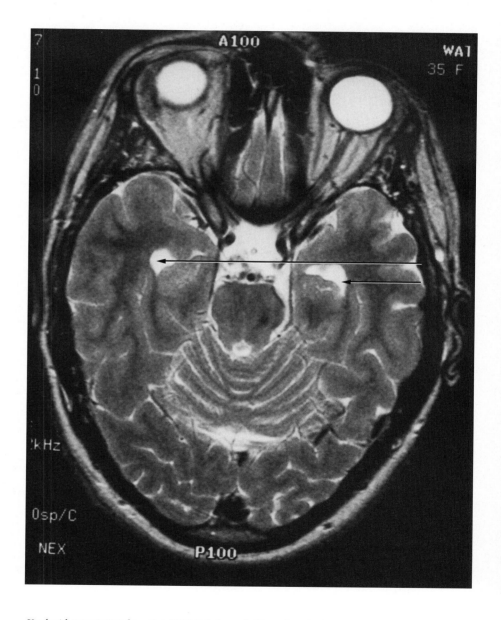

*Used with permission from Patel VH, Friedman L: Normal variations in MR imaging of the brain.*
Seminars in Ultrasound, CT, and MRI *1995;16:175–185.*

Figure **19.20**

Ventricles, lateral body, asymmetric appearance (*arrows*), axial T1-weighted image.

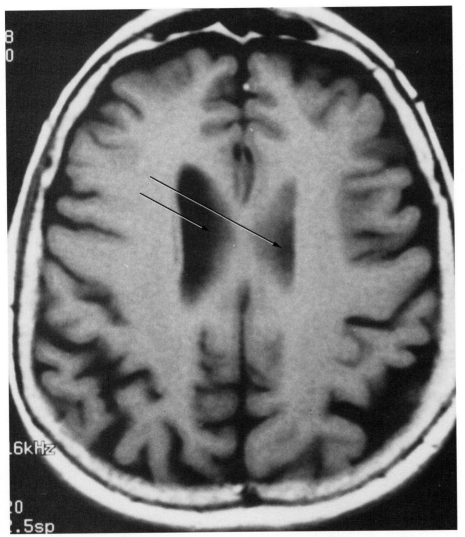

*Used with permission from Patel VH, Friedman L: Normal variations in MR imaging of the brain.* Seminars in Ultrasound, CT, and MRI *1995;16:175–185.*

## Asymmetric Body of the Lateral Ventricles
(Figures **19.20** to **19.23**)

Because of a slight tilt of the head, the CSF of the body of the lateral ventricles (Figures 19.20 and 19.21) in the high parietal images can mimic an apparently high-signal-intensity mass lesion.

Figure **19.21**

Ventricles, lateral body, asymmetric appearance
(*arrows*), axial T2-weighted image.

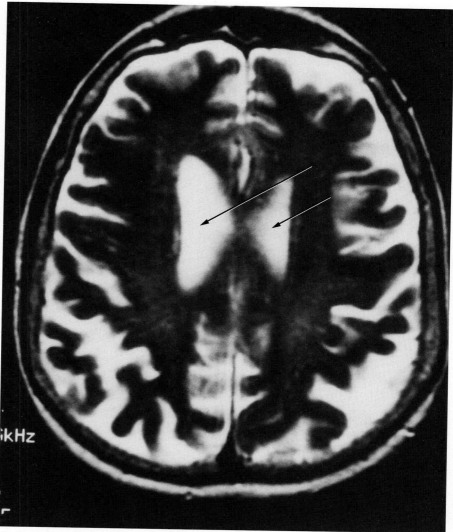

*Used with permission from Patel VH, Friedman L: Normal variations in MR imaging of the brain.*
Seminars in Ultrasound, CT, and MRI *1995;16:175–185.*

The corresponding previous image will show this asymmetricity,
thus confirming that the apparent abnormal signal corresponds to
CSF in the lateral ventricle and not a demyelinating plaque. In the
same fashion, temporal CSF (Figures 19.22 and 19.23) surrounding
the cavernous sinus (*arrows*) may mimic a high-signal mass lesion.

Figure **19.22**

Ventricles, temporal CSF (*arrows*), axial image, inverse video setting.

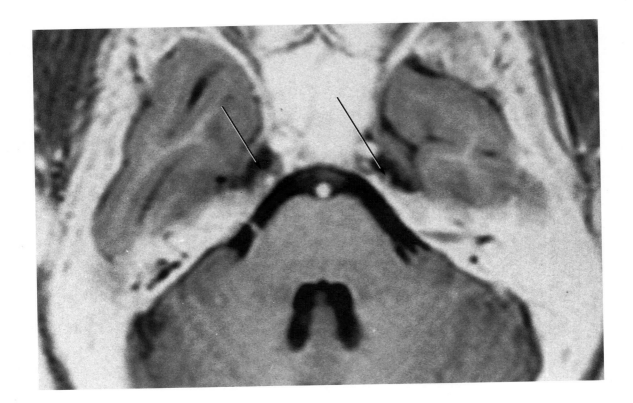

*Used with permission from Patel VH, Friedman L: Normal variations in MR imaging of the brain.* Seminars in Ultrasound, CT, and MRI *1995;16:175–185.*

Figure **19.23**

Ventricles, temporal CSF (*arrows*), axial T-2 weighted image.

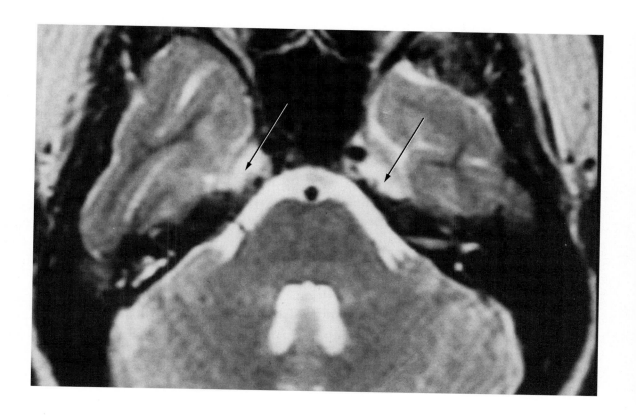

*Used with permission from Patel VH, Friedman L: Normal variations in MR imaging of the brain.* Seminars in Ultrasound, CT, and MRI *1995;16:175–185.*

## Parietal Perforators and Pseudoplaques
(Figures **19.24** to **19.27**)

*Location*:   The parietal perforators are perpendicular to the lateral ventricular system, in an orientation similar to the periventricular white matter, which is affected so commonly in multiple sclerosis.

*Appearance*:   We see the perforators as linear foci of high signal intensity (*arrows*) on T1- and T2-weighted images. Often they are of low signal intensity on T1-weighted images and of high signal intensity on T2-weighted images.

---

**N O T E**   True multiple sclerosis plaques are of high signal intensity relative to white and gray matter. The parietal perforators are not associated with atrophy or mass effects.

Note the ependymitis granularis in Figure 19.26 (*curved arrows*) and pseudolesions of the body of the lateral ventricles in Figure 19.27.

---

## Cavum Septi Pellucidi

(Also discussed with normal anatomy)

*Location*:   Between the two septal leaves.

*Appearance*:   They are CSF-filled collections between the septal leaves.

Figure **19.24**

Ventricles, parietal perforators (*arrows*),
axial magnified image.

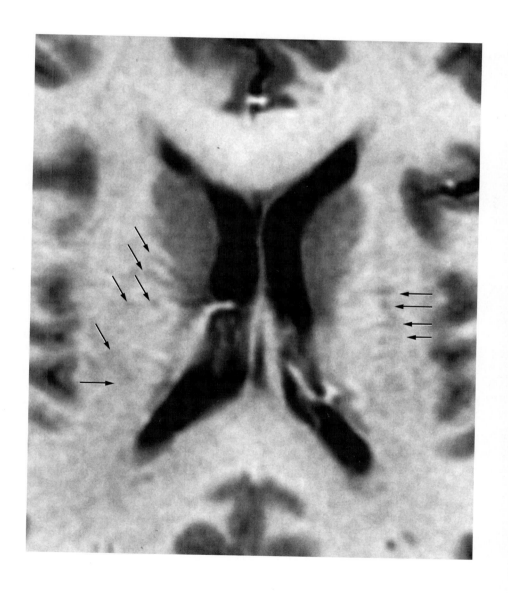

*Used with permission from Patel VH, Friedman L: Normal variations in MR imaging of the brain.*
Seminars in Ultrasound, CT, and MRI *1995;16:175–185.*

> **NOTE** The cavum septi pellucidi are present in 80 percent of normal neonates. They usually disappear after birth. However, they persist in 2 to 4 percent of normal adults and therefore are seen on CT or MRI.

## Cavum Verge

(Also discussed with normal anatomy)

*Location*:   In the midline below the corpus callosum and between the fornices.

*Appearance*:   As a CSF-filled collection seen as a posterior extension of a cavum septi pellucidi.

> **NOTE** We see the cavum verge in 30 percent of term infants. Both cavum verge and cavum septi disappear after birth. These lesions persist in 2 to 4 percent of normal adults and therefore are seen on CT or MRI. Cavum verge never occurs without cavum septi.

Figure **19.25**

Ventricles, parietal perforators (*arrows*), axial magnified image.

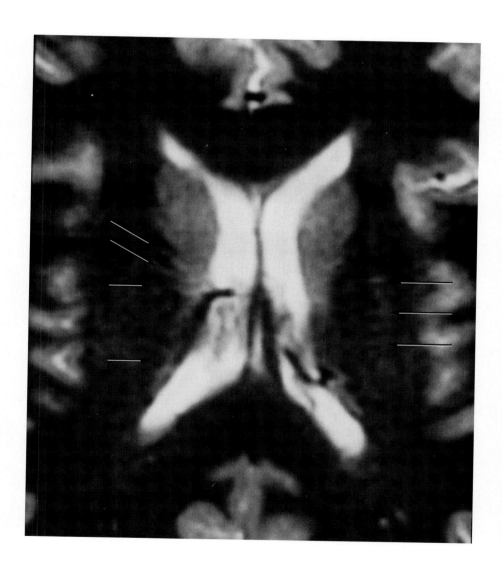

Figure **19.26**

Ventricles, parietal perforators (*small arrows*), axial proton density image.

Ependymitis granularis

Parietal perforators

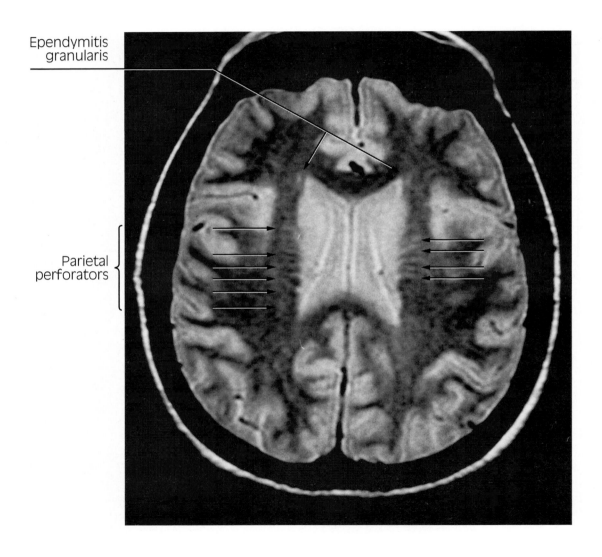

Figure **19.27**

Ventricles, parietal perforators (*small arrows*), axial T2-weighted image.

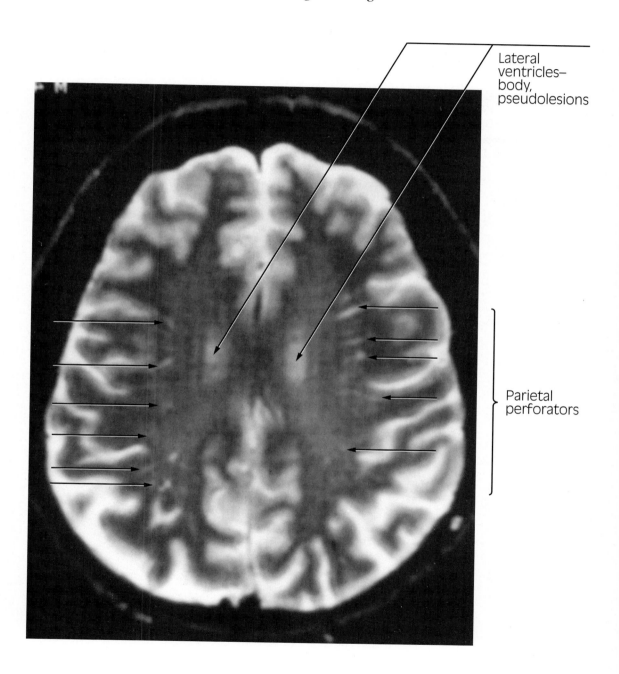

Lateral ventricles– body, pseudolesions

Parietal perforators

## Brain Stem

### Red Nucleus
(Figure **19.28**)

*Location*:   Centrally in the midbrain or mesencephalon.

*Appearance*:   We see the red nucleus as an area of low signal intensity on sagittal T1-weighted and proton density images centrally in the midbrain. It should not be mistaken for being pathological.

> **N O T E**   The low signal is due to the iron content. Depending upon how much iron content is present in this region, hypointensity is variable on T2-weighted images. In this figure, also note the normal high signal of the posterior pituitary gland.
>
> We also characteristically see this low signal pattern in the globus pallidus and pars reticulum of the substantia nigra on T1- and T2-weighted images.

Figure **19.28**

Brain stem, red nucleus,
sagittal T1-weighted image.

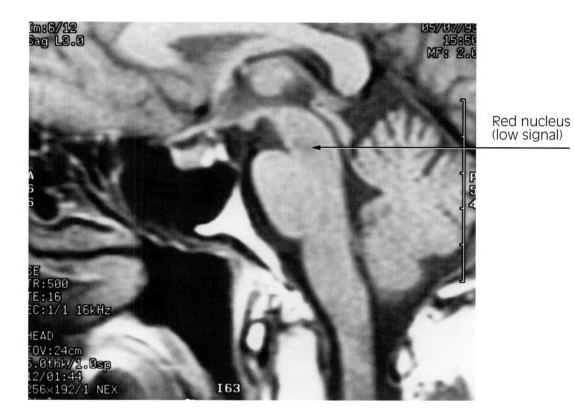

Red nucleus
(low signal)

## Corticospinal Hyperintensity

*Location*: Lateral aspect of the lower pons (Figures **19.29** and **19.30**).

Lateral aspect of the upper pons (Figures **19.31** and **19.32**).

Lateral aspect of the cerebral peduncles (Figures **19.33** and **19.34**), just anterior to the substantia nigra

*Appearance*: We see the corticospinal tracts as an asymmetric or symmetric punctate area of high or low signal intensity on both T1- and T2-weighted images.

---

**N O T E** We should not mistake this pattern of the corticospinal tracts for lacunar infarcts. True lacunar infarcts are associated with atrophy, a decrease in peduncular size, or gliosis.

---

## Medullary Claval Pseudotumor
(Figures **19.35** to **19.37**)

*Location*: Posterior inferior medulla or myelencephalon.

*Appearance*: A protrusion or elevation of the posterior inferior portion of the medulla.

---

**N O T E** The medullary claval pseudotumor is seen as a protrusion from the posterior and inferior surface of the medulla. This area houses the nucleus cuneatus and gracilis and appears prominent in most normal individuals. Recognizing its iso-signal intensity as similar to the remaining brain stem on multiple imaging sequences is important. Note the normal low signal intensity of the substantia nigra in Figures 19.35 and 19.36. Also, note thinning of the body of the corpus callosum as a normal variant in Figure 19.37.

Figure **19.29**

Brain stem, lower pons, cortical tracts, axial image.

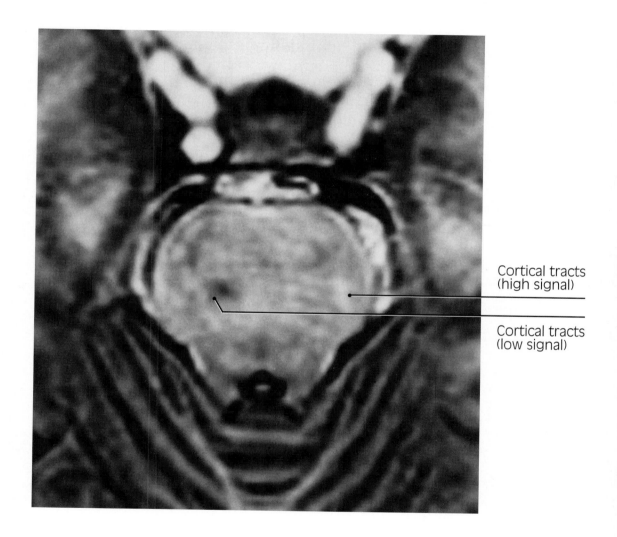

Cortical tracts
(high signal)

Cortical tracts
(low signal)

Figure **19.30**

Brain stem, lower pons, cortical tracts, axial image.

Cortical tracts
(low signal)

Cortical tracts
(bright signal)

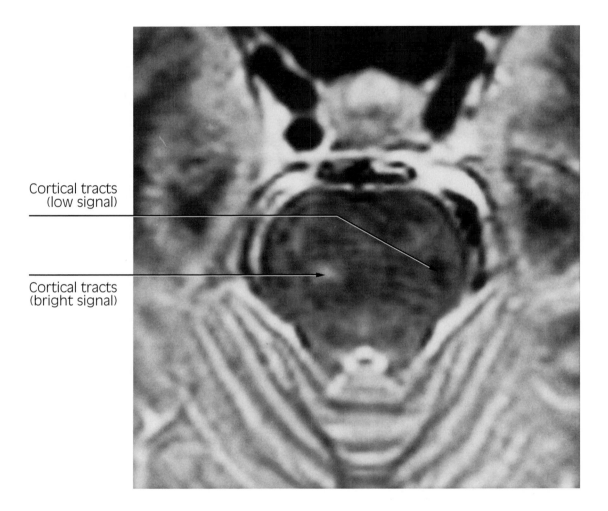

Figure **19.31**

Brain stem, upper pons, cortical tracts,
sagittal image.

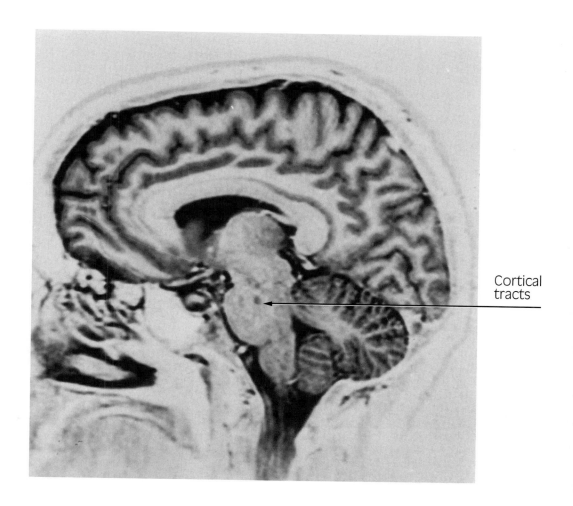

Cortical
tracts

Figure **19.32**

Brain stem, upper pons, cortical tracts, sagittal image.

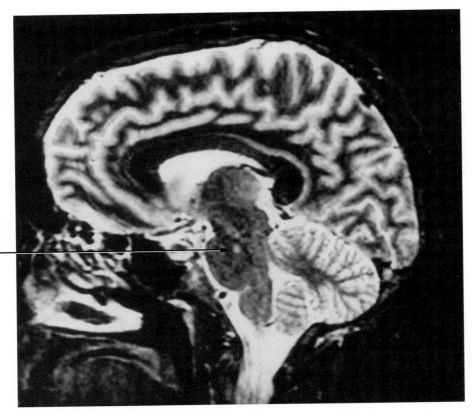

Cortical
tracts

Figure **19.33**

Brain stem, cerebral peduncles, corticospinal tract,
axial image.

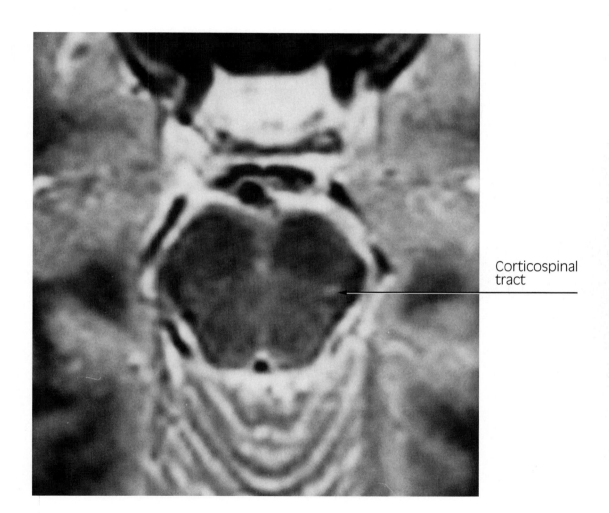

Corticospinal
tract

Figure **19.34**

Brain stem, cerebral peduncles, corticospinal tract, axial image.

Corticospinal
tract

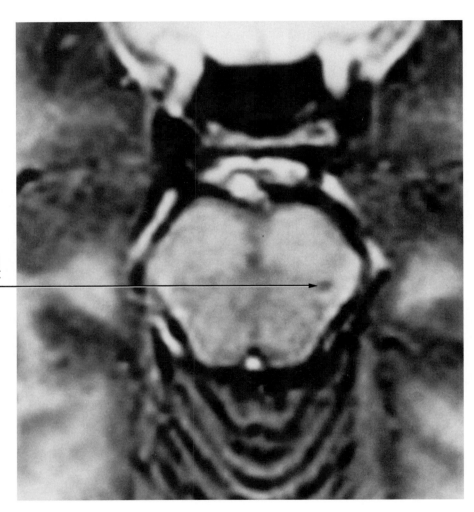

Figure **19.35**

Brain stem, medullary claval pseudotumor,
sagittal image.

Substantia
nigra (low
signal)

Medullary
claval
pseudotumor

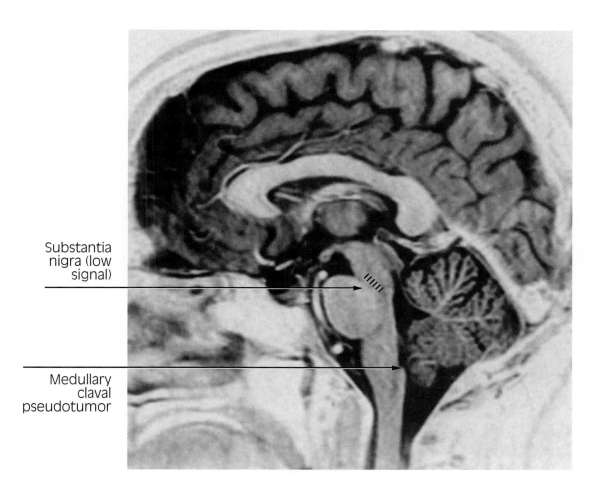

Figure **19.36**

Brain stem, medullary claval pseudotumor, sagittal image.

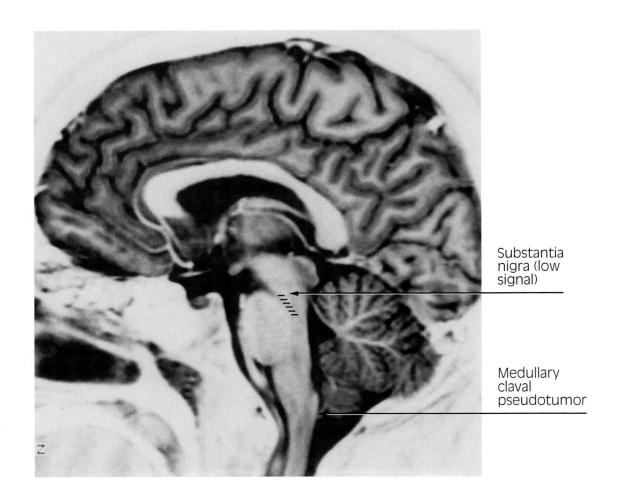

Substantia nigra (low signal)

Medullary claval pseudotumor

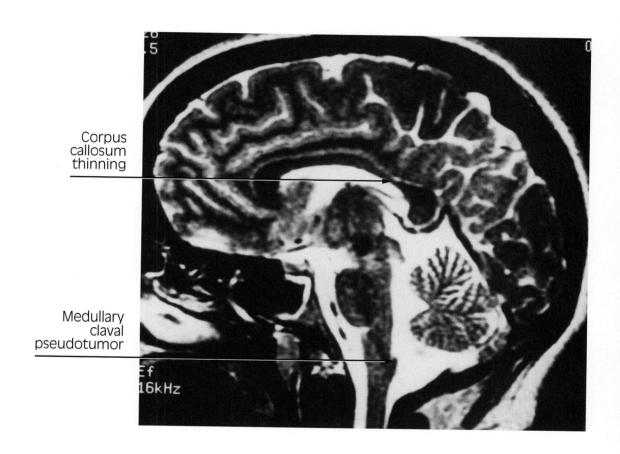

Figure **19.37**

Brain stem, medullary claval pseudotumor,
sagittal T2-weighted image.

Corpus
callosum
thinning

Medullary
claval
pseudotumor

# Cranial Nerves

## Pseudolesions of the Optic Nerve
(Figure **19.38**)

CSF surrounding the optic nerves on T2-weighted images, including fat-saturated sequences, should not be mistaken for optic neuritis.

## Lateral Displacement of the Optic Nerve
(Figures **19.39** to **19.42**)

Figures 19.39 and 19.40, coronal images show lateral displacement of the left optic nerve. The corresponding axial images do not show any mass lesion displacing the left optic nerve. The pseudo-displacement of the optic nerve occurs because of more prominent but normal retrobulbar fat.

Figure **19.38**

Cranial nerves, optic nerve pseudolesions, (CSF), axial T2-weighted image.

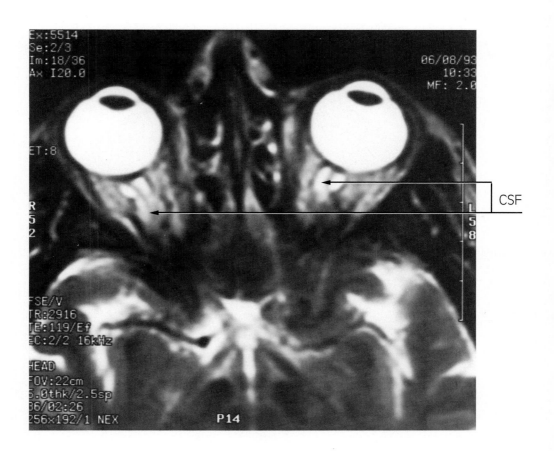

Figure **19.39**

Cranial nerves, optic nerve (lateral displacement), coronal image.

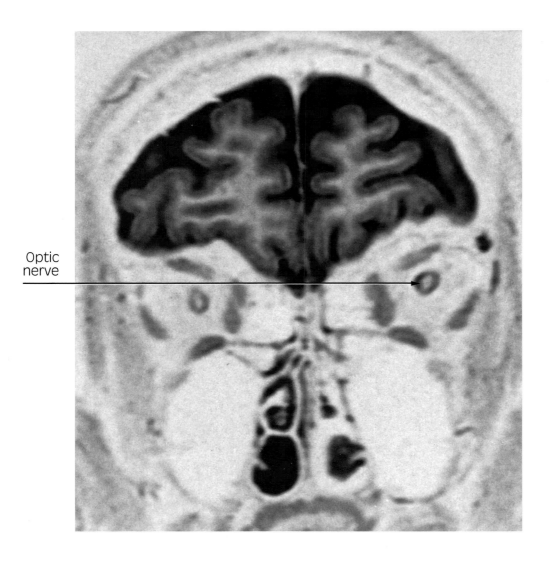

Optic nerve

Figure **19.40**

Cranial nerves, optic nerve (lateral displacement), coronal T2-weighted image.

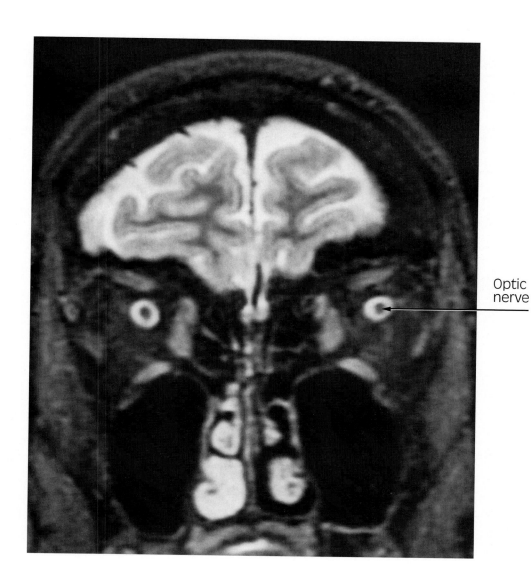

Optic nerve

Figure **19.41**

Cranial nerves, optic nerve (lateral displacement), axial T1-weighted image.

Optic
nerve

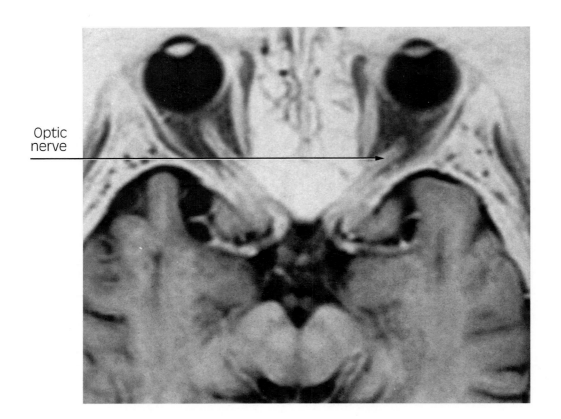

Figure **19.42**

Cranial nerves, optic nerve (lateral displacement),
axial T2-weighted image.

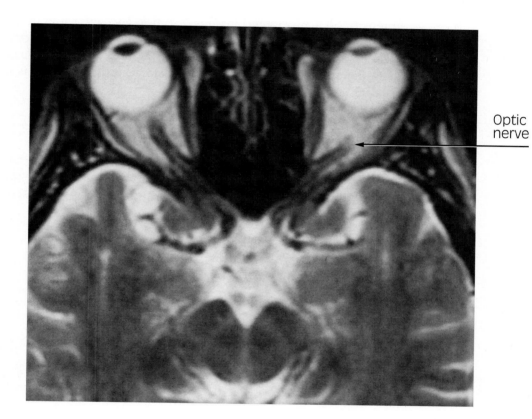

Optic
nerve

## Vascular Structures

### Virchow-Robin Spaces
(Figures **19.43** and **19.44**)

Perivascular Virchow-Robin spaces normally surround perforating arteries that enter the medial temporal lobes, corpus striatum, and thalami. Their characteristic low signal intensity on T1-weighted images, isointensity with CSF on proton density images, high signal intensity on T2-weighted images, location (not infrequently in the region of the basal ganglia), and relationship with the perforating arteries distinguish them from lacunar infarcts, cystic neoplasms, or parasitic cysts. In the past we misinterpreted these spaces as lacunar infarcts in young patients on CT.

### Jugular Foramen
(Figure **19.45**)

Slow flow in the internal jugular vein or fatty tissue in the pars vascularis of the jugular foramen appears as hyperintensity on axial T1-weighted images and can simulate thrombosis of the internal jugular vein.

Figure **19.43**

Virchow-Robin spaces,
axial T1-weighted image.

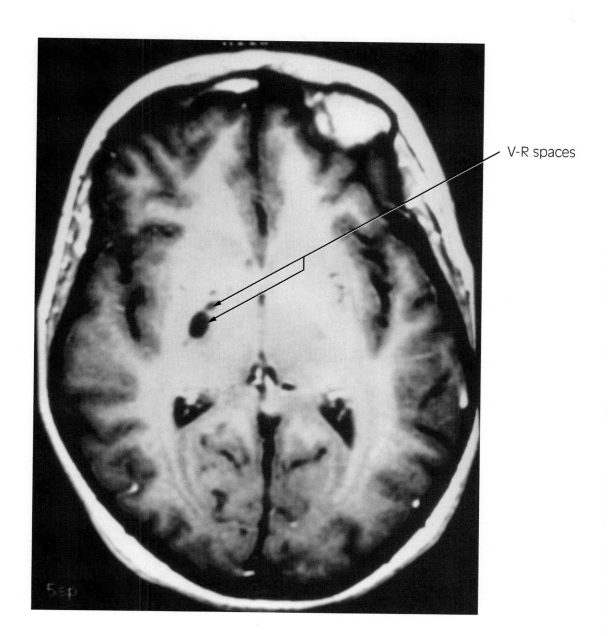

V-R spaces

Figure **19.44**

Virchow-Robin spaces, axial T2-weighted image.

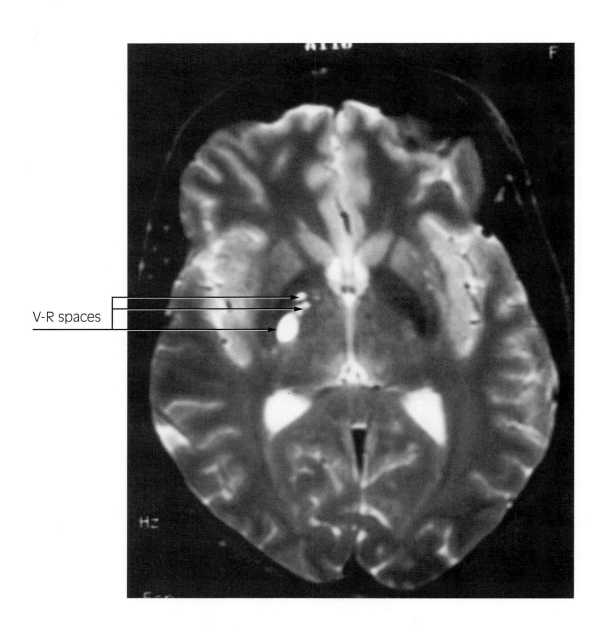

Figure **19.45**

Jugular foramen, axial T1-weighted image.

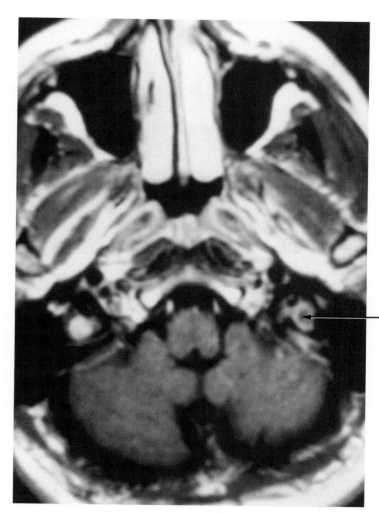

Internal jugular vein (slow flow)

## Ectatic Basilar Artery
(Figures **19.46** and **19.47**)

These figures show an ectatic basilar artery and a prominent but normal lateral medullary cistern, causing a mass effect on the left lateral and superior portion of the medulla.

## Lateral Ventricle Pseudocystic Mass Lesion
(Figure **19.48**)

This figure shows a spurious cystic-appearing lesion with a peripheral bright rim in the body of the right lateral ventricle. This uncommon variation occurs as a result of (a) partial volume averaging from the flow void signal of the neighboring vessel projecting into the body of the lateral ventricle, or (b) partial volume averaging from the neighboring normal choroid plexus or its small cyst projecting through the lateral ventricle, or (c) both. This variation mimics an intraventricular lesion such as a tumor, cysticercosis, or a tuberculoma.

## Anterior Cerebral Artery Hypoplasia and Narrowing
(Figures **19.49** and **19.50**)

Time-of-flight MR arterial angiogram through the circle of Willis shows narrowing of the A1 segment of the left anterior cerebral artery (ACA). Note that there is no evidence of intraluminal disease.

Figure **19.46**

Ectatic basilar artery,
axial T1-weighted image.

Basilar
artery

Lateral
medullary
cistern

Medulla

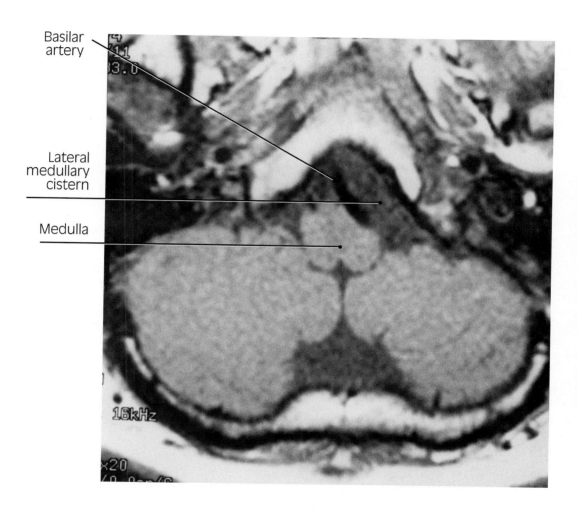

Figure **19.47**

Ectatic basilar artery,
axial T2-weighted image.

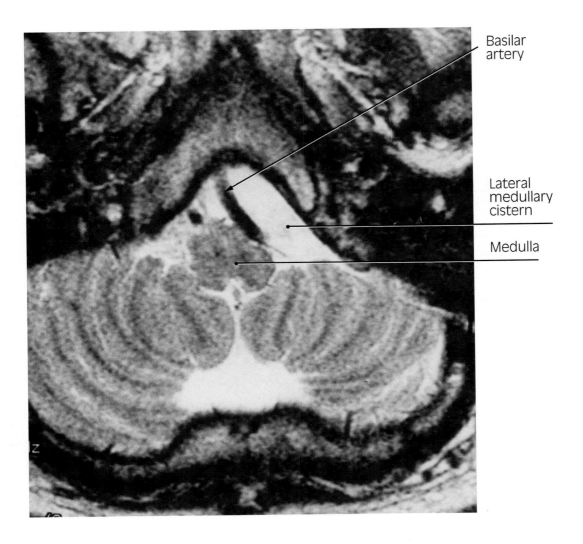

Basilar
artery

Lateral
medullary
cistern

Medulla

Figure **19.48**

Lateral ventricle pseudolesion,
axial proton density image.

Pseudocystic
lesion

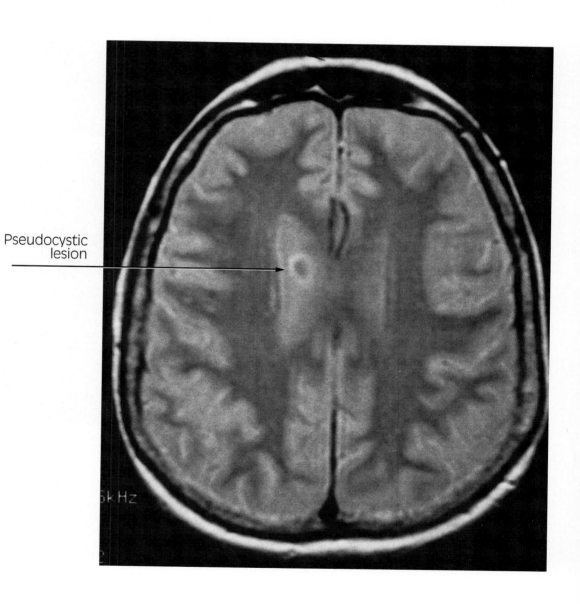

Figure **19.49**

Hypoplasia and narrowing of ACA,
time-of-flight MR arterial angiogram.

Left ACA,
A1 segment

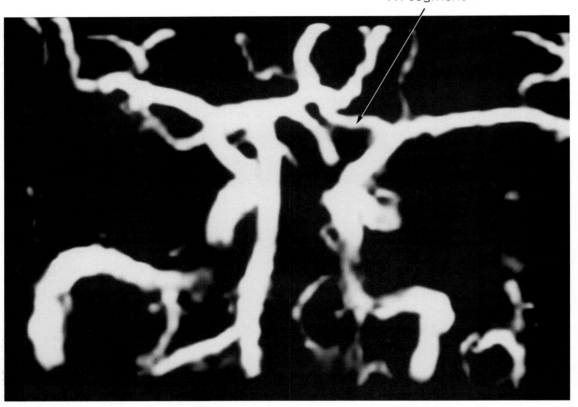

Figure **19.50**

Hypoplasia and narrowing of ACA,
time-of-flight MR arterial angiogram.

Left ACA,
A1 segment

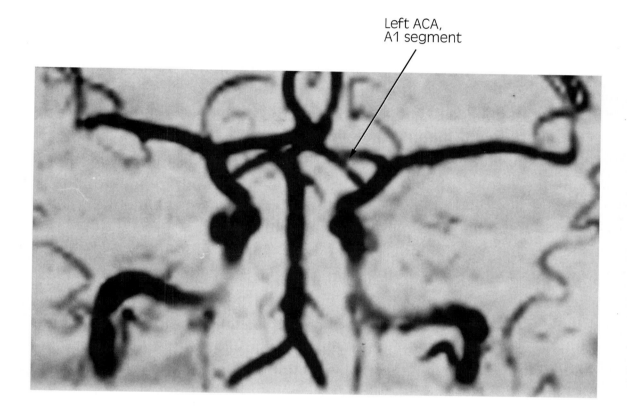

# Pituitary Gland and Sella

### Empty Sella
(Figures **19.51** and **19.52**)

This refers to as anatomic finding of a severely flattened pituitary gland due to a primary deficiency of the diaphragmatic sella resulting in an enlarged diaphragmatic hiatus. The superior portion of the sella that appears "empty" on T1-weighted images is filled with CSF. Symptoms are rare. Most frequently we see this as an incidental finding of little or no clinical significance.

### Anterior Pituitary, Low Signal
(Figures **19.53** and **19.54**)

Partial volume averaging from the cavernous internal carotid artery results in an apparently low-signal mass lesion in the anterior pituitary.

### Pituitary Stalk or Infundibulum
(Figures **19.55** and **19.56**)

We should not misinterpret the centrally located bright pituitary stalk on axial T1-weighted images for being abnormal.

### Bright Posterior Pituitary
(Figures **19.57** to **19.60**)

The high signal intensity of the posterior pituitary on T1-weighted images (Figure **19.57**) is one of the most common normal variations in MRI of the brain. There may be more than one source of this high-intensity signal, but in most cases neurosecretory vesicles seem responsible. We also commonly see the bright posterior pituitary in neonates (Figures **19.58** to **19.60**) and in the pediatric age group.

### Posterior Pituitary, Absent Bright Signal
(Figure **19.61**)

Absence of the normal high-intensity signal in the posterior pituitary gland on T1-weighted images can be a normal variant in asymptomatic individuals. Compare with normal high signal intensity in this area in Figure 19.57.

---

**NOTE** Absent high signal of the posterior pituitary is often, but not invariably, associated with central diabetes insipidus or compressive pituitary gland lesions.

Figure **19.51**

Empty sella, sagittal T1-weighted image.

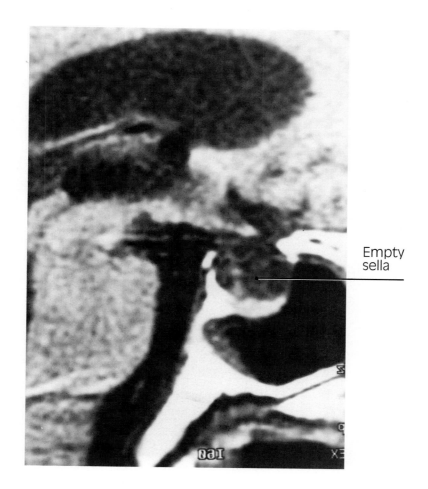

Empty
sella

Figure **19.52**

Empty sella, coronal T1-weighted image.

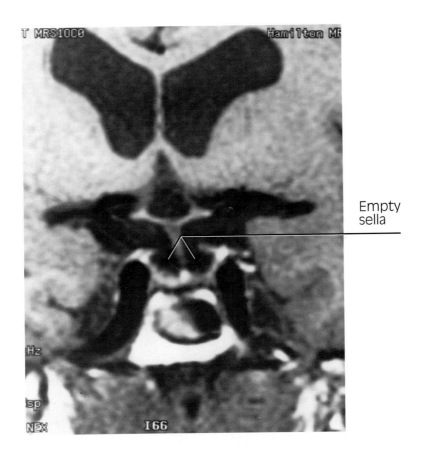

Empty
sella

Figure **19.53**

Pituitary gland, anterior pituitary, sagittal T1-weighted image.

Low signal, anterior lobe

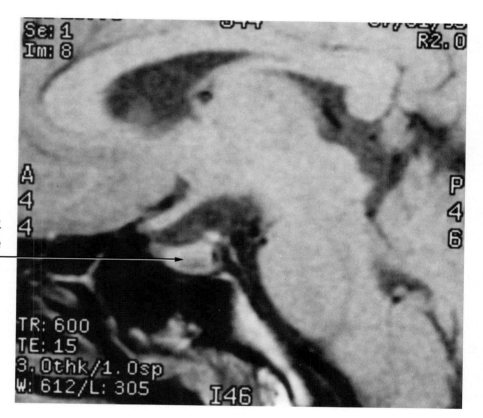

Figure **19.54**

Pituitary gland, anterior pituitary,
sagittal T1-weighted image.

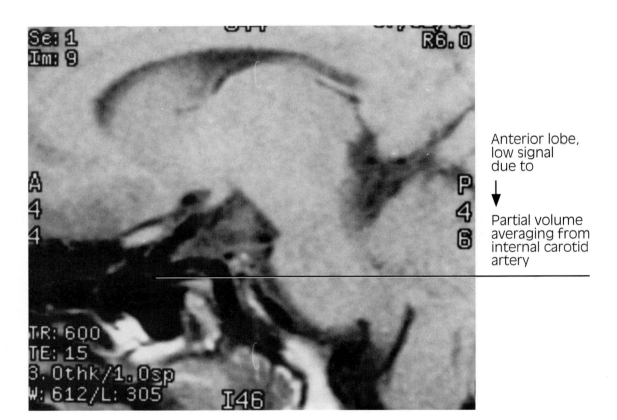

Anterior lobe,
low signal
due to

↓

Partial volume
averaging from
internal carotid
artery

Figure **19.55**

Pituitary gland, infundibulum,
axial T1-weighted image.

Infundibulum/
stalk (bright
signal)

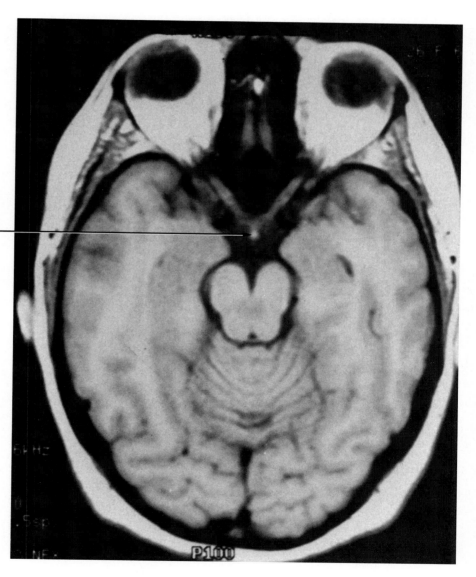

Figure **19.56**

Pituitary gland, infundibulum,
axial T1-weighted image.

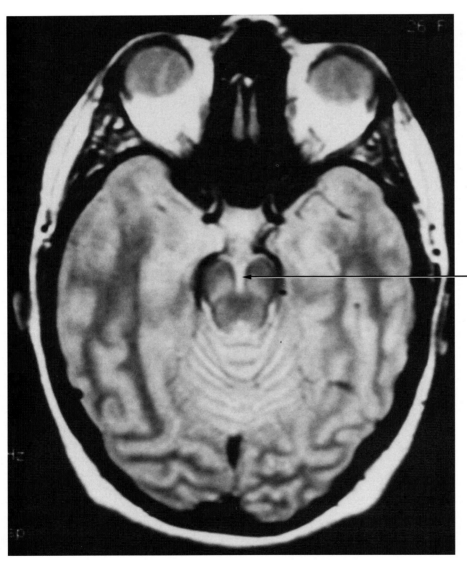

Infundibulum/
stalk

Figure **19.57**

Adult pituitary gland, posterior pituitary,
sagittal T1-weighted image.

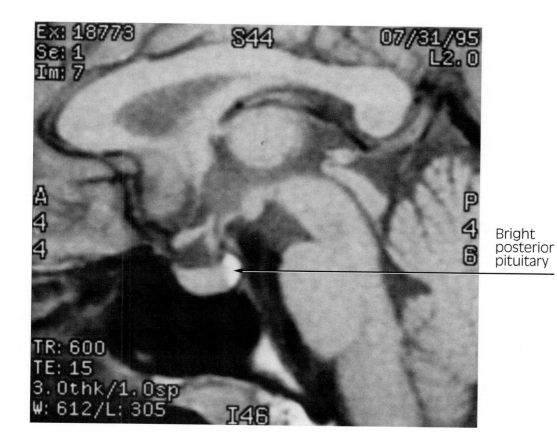

Bright
posterior
pituitary

Figure **19.58**

Neonatal pituitary gland, posterior pituitary, axial T1-weighted image.

Bright
posterior
pituitary

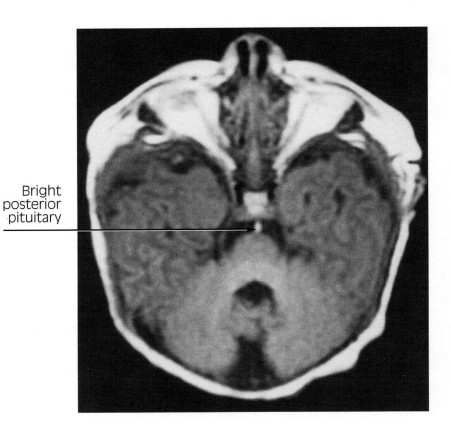

Figure **19.59**

Neonatal pituitary gland, posterior pituitary, sagittal T1-weighted image.

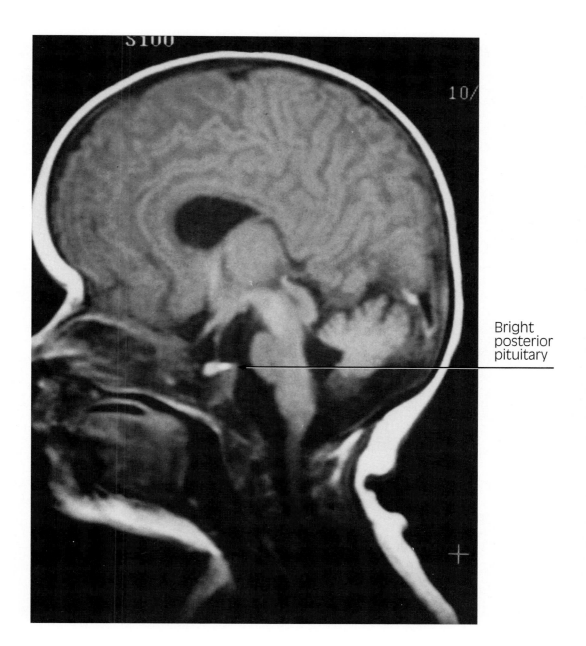

Bright posterior pituitary

Figure **19.60**

Neonatal pituitary gland, posterior pituitary, sagittal T1-weighted image, magnified.

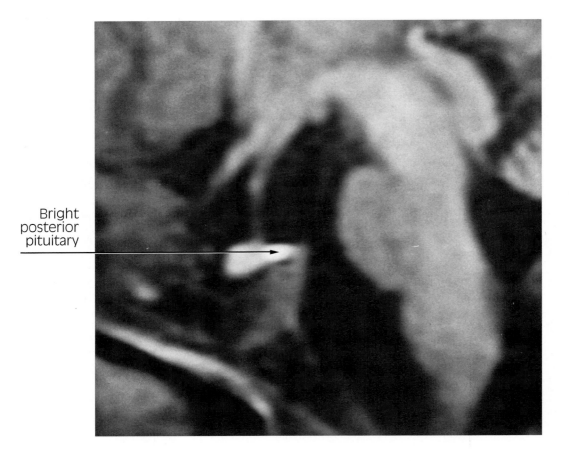

Bright
posterior
pituitary

Figure **19.61**

Pituitary gland, posterior pituitary,
sagittal T1-weighted image.

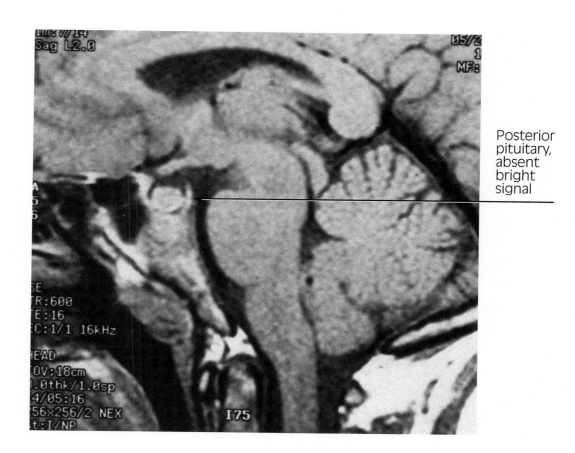

Posterior
pituitary,
absent
bright
signal

Figure **19.62**

Ectopic pituitary gland (*arrow*), coronal T1-weighted image.

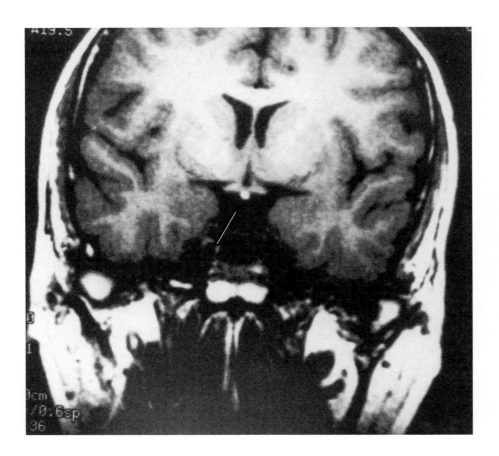

### Ectopic Posterior Pituitary
(Figures **19.62** and **19.63**)

Another important "congenital" anomaly encountered is the ectopic posterior pituitary.

*Location*:  Tuber cinereum of the hypothalamus.

*Findings*:  A small anterior pituitary and sella turcica, absence of the usual high-signal posterior pituitary, and the presence of an anomalous high-signal area in the tuber cinereum of the hypothalamus (*arrow*) on T1-weighted images.

Figure **19.63**

Ectopic pituitary gland (*arrow*),
sagittal T1-weighted image.

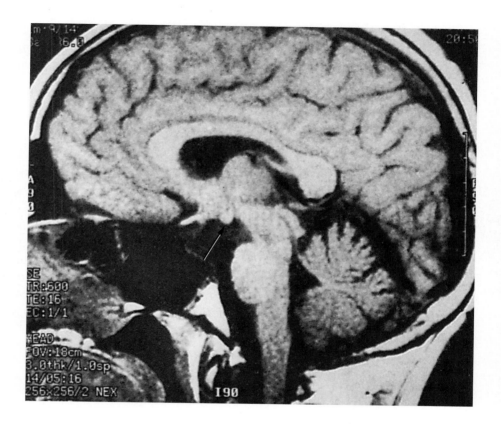

**N O T E**  Most patients with an ectopic posterior pituitary have a
history of breech or traumatic deliveries. Birth "trauma" is
thought to cause rupture of the pituitary infundibulum with
its vascular supply as the stalk is stretched between the fixed
pituitary gland and the more mobile brain. This ectopic
region functions as a posterior lobe.

# Skull Base

## Marrow Pseudolesions at Base of the Cranium
(Figure **19.64**)

An asymmetrical high-intensity signal on T1-weighted images from fatty marrow in the base of the cranium (petrous bone) may simulate lipoma, dermoid, or thrombus within vessels.

> **N O T E** This finding can also apply to the anterior clinoids, the diploic spaces, the apex of the C2 vertebra, the crista galli, the falx, the foramen magnum, and the mastoids.

## Clivus Pseudolesions
(Figures **19.65** to **19.68**)

The signal from clivus marrow is age-related and changes from uniformly low in children to uniformly high signal by age 24. Variations commonly occur, and in the third decade only 30 percent of patients may display the normal uniform high-signal pattern. As a rule, signal intensity in the clivus lower than that of the pons should be considered as abnormal, whereas uniform bright signal in the clivus is unlikely to be abnormal. Figures 19.65 and 19.66 show the variability of yellow marrow signal in the basisphenoid. Normal innominate synchondrosis in a young child is demonstrated. Signal void is also seen in the pneumatized clivus.

Figure **19.64**

Skull base, marrow pseudolesion,
axial T1-weighted image.

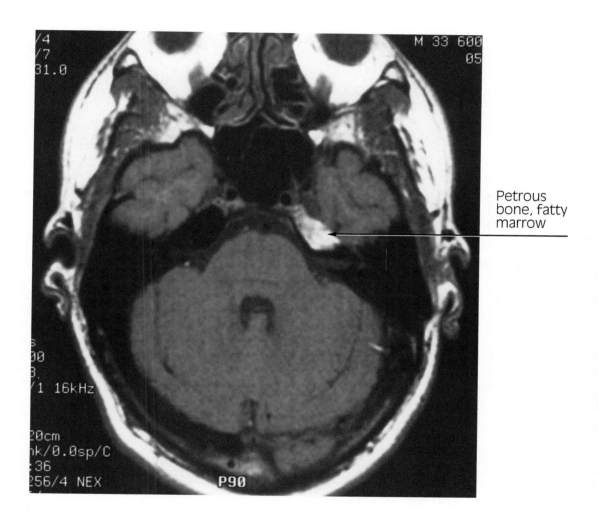

Petrous
bone, fatty
marrow

Figure **19.65**

Clivus pseudolesions,
sagittal T1-weighted image.

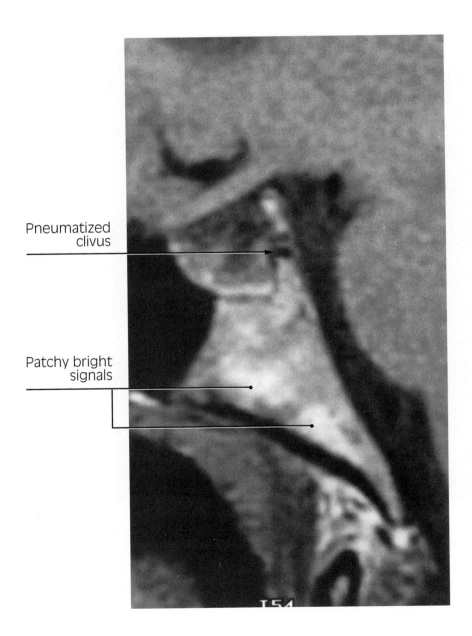

Pneumatized
clivus

Patchy bright
signals

Figure **19.66**

Clivus pseudolesions,
sagittal T1-weighted image.

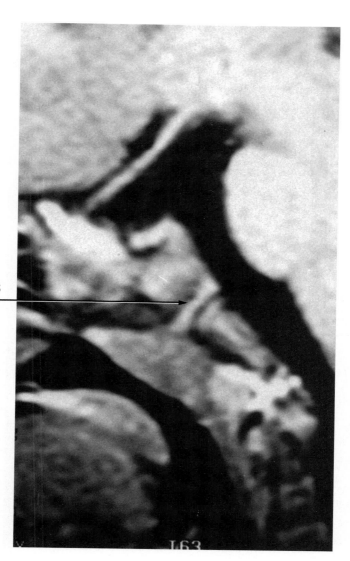

Synchondrosis

Figure **19.67**

Clivus pseudolesions,
axial T1-weighted image.

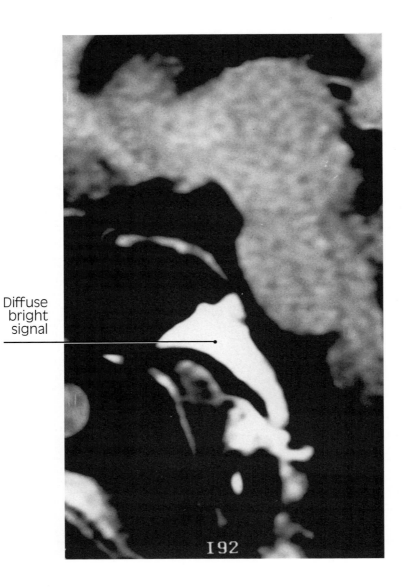

Diffuse
bright
signal

Figure **19.68**

Clivus pseudolesions,
sagittal T1-weighted image.

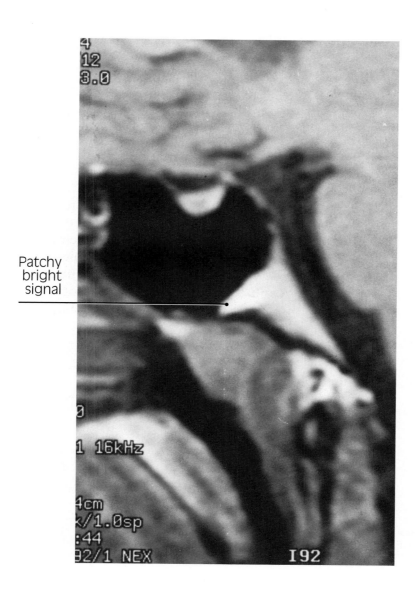

Patchy
bright
signal

## Paranasal Sinuses and Mastoids
(Figure **19.69**)

We should recognize incidental mucosal thickening and polyps in the sinuses and not mistake them for more sinister pathology. A sphenoid polyp is shown in Figure 19.13, and left mastoid mucosal changes are illustrated in Figure 19.69.

## Miscellaneous

### Pineal Gland Cysts
(Figure **19.70**)

Small asymptomatic nonneoplastic pineal gland cysts are common incidental findings, seen in up to 40 percent of routine autopsies and in 1 to 5 percent of unselected MRI scans.

> **NOTE** Pineal gland cysts occur because of degenerative change, coalescence of small cysts, sequestration of a pineal diverticulum, and failure of normal pineal development. Occasionally, the imaging appearance of a benign pineal cyst is indistinguishable from that of small cystic pineal neoplasms such as pineocytomas. CT- or MR-guided stereotactic biopsy has been recommended for the evaluation and management of symptomatic cases.

### Neuroepithelial or Neuroglial Cysts
#### Choroid Plexus Cysts
(Figure **19.71**)

A gadolinium contrast–enhanced axial T1-weighted image shows nonenhancing, multiple bilateral, well-defined simple cysts of the choroid plexus.

> **NOTE** Most symptomatic neuroepithelial cysts in the lateral ventricle are found in the trigone.

Figure **19.69**

Mastoid, mucosal thickening,
axial T2-weighted image.

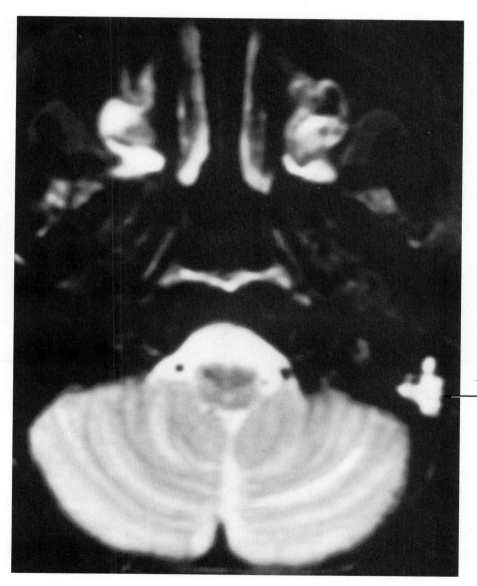

Mucosal
thickening

Figure **19.70**

Pineal gland cyst,
sagittal T1-weighted image.

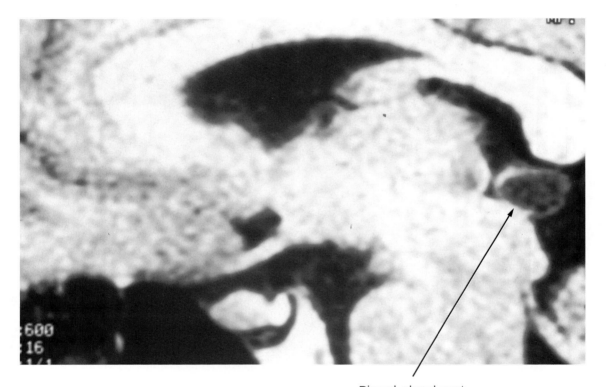

Pineal gland cyst

Figure **19.71**

Choroid plexus cysts, axial T1-weighted image, after contrast.

Choroid plexus cysts

Choroid plexus cysts

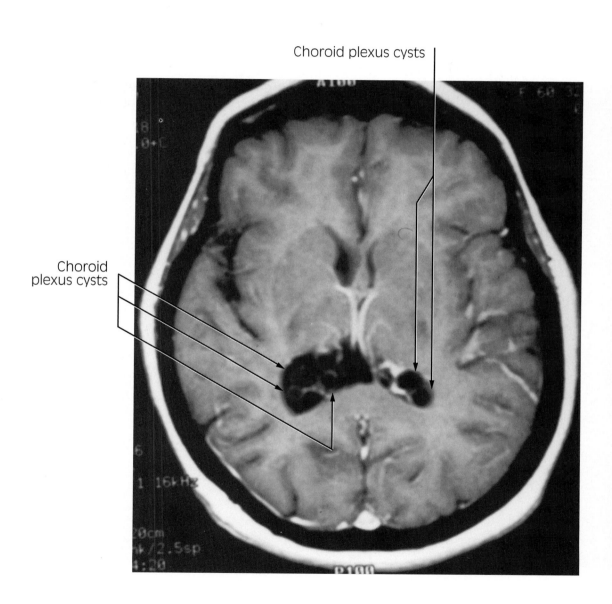

## Choroid Fissure Cysts
(Figures **19.72** to **19.74**)

The choroid fissure cyst is an ovoid or spindle-shaped nonenhancing CSF-like cyst commonly seen at the medial temporal lobe between the hippocampus and the diencephalon.

> **N O T E**  The choroidal fissure is a CSF space between the fimbria of the hippocampus and the diencephalon that curves posterosuperiorly from the anterior temporal lobe to the atrium of the lateral ventricle.

Figure **19.72**

Choroid fissure cyst,
coronal precontrast image.

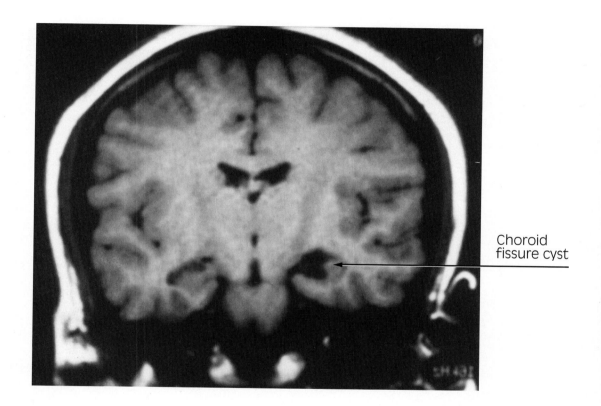

Choroid
fissure cyst

Figure **19.73**

Choroid fissure cyst,
axial precontrast image.

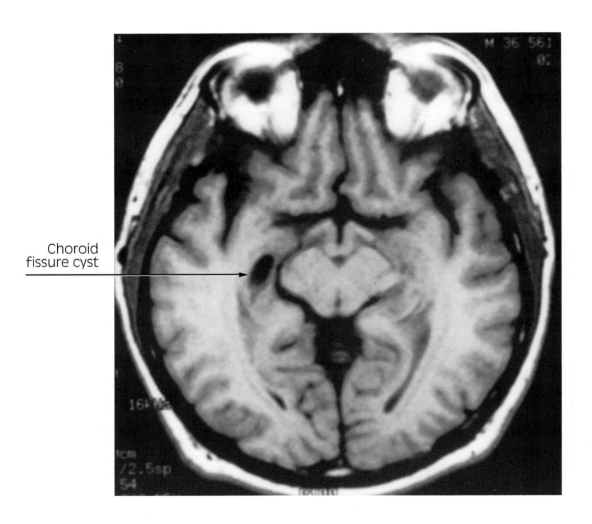

Choroid
fissure cyst

Figure **19.74**

Choroid fissure cyst, axial postcontrast image.

Choroid
fissure cyst

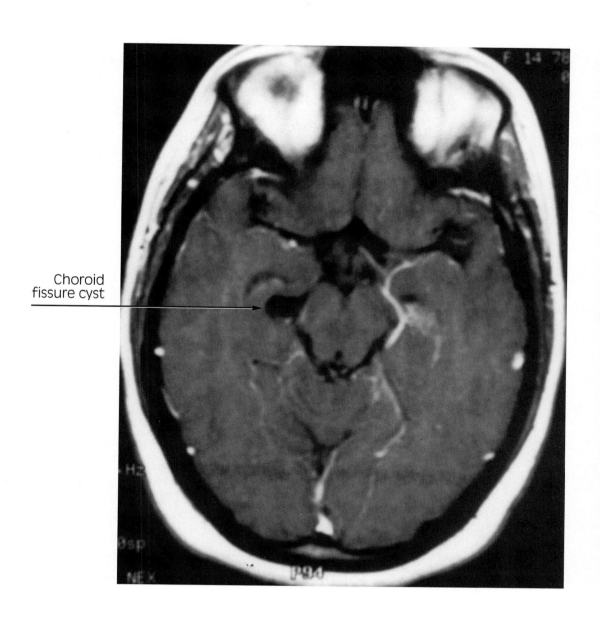

# Bibliography

Atlas S, ed: *Magnetic Resonance Imaging of the Brain and Spine*. Philadelphia: Lippincott–Raven, 1996.

Berry M, Standring SM, Bannister LH. Nervous system. In William PL, ed: *Gray's Anatomy: The Anatomical Basis of Medicine and Surgery*. New York: Churchill Livingstone, 1995; 901.

Bjorklund A, Hokfelt T, Wouterlood FG, et al., eds: *Handbook of Chemical Neuroanatomy*. Amsterdam: Elsevier, 1990.

Chusid JG, ed: *Correlative Neuroanatomy and Functional Neurology*. Los Altos: Lange Medical Publications, 1985.

Friedman L, Patel VH. Normal variations in MR imaging of the brain. *Seminars in Ultrasound, CT, and MRI* 1995;16:175–185.

Jones EG, ed: *The Thalamus*. New York: Plenum Press, 1985.

Lourie JA, ed: *Medical Eponyms*. London: Pitman Pub. Ltd., 1983.

Neurologic disorders. In Isselbacher KJ, Braunwald E, Wilson JD, et al., eds: *Harrison's Principles of Internal Medicine*. 13th ed. New York: McGraw-Hill, 1994.

Ono M, Kubik S, Abernathy CD, eds: *Atlas of the Cerebral Sulci*. New York: George Thieme Verlag and Thieme Medical Publishers, Inc., 1990.

Osborn AG, ed: *Diagnostic Neuroradiology*. St. Louis: Mosby, 1994.

Patel VH, Friedman L. MR imaging of the brain: Normal anatomy. A teaching exercise. *Radiographics Neuroradiology CD-ROM* 1995;15:24.

Schnitzlein HN, Reed Murtagh F, et al. *Imaging Anatomy of the Head and Spine*. Baltimore-Munich: Urban & Schwarzenberg, 1985.

Swash M, Oxbury J, eds: *Clinical Neurology, Volume I and II*. Edinburgh: Churchill Livingstone, 1991.

Taveras JM, ed: *Neuroradiology*. Baltimore: Williams & Wilkins, 1996.

Waddington MM, eds: *Atlas of Human Intracranial Anatomy*. Vermont: Academy Books, 1984.

Weir J, Abrahams PH, Belli A-M, eds: *Imaging Atlas of Human Anatomy*. Aylesbury, England: Mosby–Year Book Europe Ltd. and Wolfe Pub. Ltd., 1992.

# Glossary
## of Important Names in Neurology and Neuroradiology

**Alzheimer, Alois** (1864–1915); clinical neurologist and pathologist, Frankfurt
> Alzheimer's disease: a form of presenile dementia, diagnosed in 1906

**Arnold, Julius A.** (1835–1915); professor of pathological anatomy, Heidelberg
> Arnold-Chiari malformation: hindbrain anomaly, diagnosed in 1894

**Berry, Sir James** (1860–1946); surgeon, Canada
> Berry's aneurysm: its rupture may be the cause of a subarachnoid hemorrhage

**Broca, Pierre Paul** (1824–1880); professor of clinical surgery, Paris
> Broca's speech area: in the cerebral cortex, diagnosed in 1861

**Brodmann, Korbinian** (1868–1918); neurologist, Germany
> Brodmann's areas of the cerebral cortex

**Charcot, Jean-Martin** (1825–1893); professor of pathological anatomy, Paris
> Charcot's lenticulostriate artery of cerebral hemorrhage
> Maladie de Charcot: motor neuron disease

**von Chiari, Hans** (1851–1916); professor of pathological anatomy, Strasbourg and Prague
> Arnold-Chiari malformation

**Cushing, Harvey Williams** (1869–1939); "Founder of Neurosurgery," United States and France
> Cushing's syndrome of adult hyperadrenocorticism: diagnosed in 1932
> Described the pituitary gland as "the conductor of the endocrine orchestra"

**Edinger, Ludwig** (1855–1918); professor of neurology, Goethe University, Frankfurt
> Edinger-Westphal nucleus of the oculomotor nerve: concerned with accommodation, diagnosed in 1885

**Galen, Claudius** (AD 130–200); surgeon, Pergamum; top physician, Venice
> Great vein of Galen

**Ganser, Sigbert Joseph Maria** (1853–1931); psychiatrist, Dresden
> Ganser's hypothalamic commissure

**Giacomini, Carlo** (1841–1898); anatomist, Italy
> Giacomini's band of the dentate gyrus

**Gubler, Adolphe Marie** (1821–1879); physician, France
> Millard-Gubler syndrome

**Gudden, Bernhard Alloys** (1824–1886); neurologist, Germany
> Gudden's supraoptic commissure

**Herschl, Richard L.** (1824–1881); pathologist, Austria
> Herschl's gyrus

**Huntington, George** (1850–1916); physician, Ohio, North Carolina, and New York
> Huntington's chorea: diagnosed in 1972

**Labbe, Leon** (1832–1916); surgeon, France
> Vein of Labbe

**Lancisi, Giovanni Maria** (1654–1720); physician, Italy
> Lancisi's medical and lateral longitudinal striae

**von Luschka, Hubert** (1820–1875); professor of anatomy, Tubingen
> Foramen of Luschka: in the lateral recess of the fourth ventricle, diagnosed in 1855

**Luys, Jules Bernard** (1828–1897); physician, France
> Luys' nucleus subthalamicus

**Millard, Auguste L. J.** (1830–1915); physician, France
> Millard-Gubler syndrome

**Megendie, Francois** (1783–1855); professor of medicine, pathology, and physiology, France
  Foramen of Megendie: medical opening in the fourth ventricle, diagnosed in 1828

**Meckel, Johann Friedrich I** (1714–1774); professor of anatomy, botany, and gynecology, Berlin
  Meckel's cave and ganglion

**Meynert, Theodor Herman** (1833–1892); professor of neurology and psychiatry, Vienna
  Meynert's supraoptic commissure

**Monro, Alexander** (1733–1817); professor of anatomy, Edinburgh
  Foramen of Monro: interventricular foramen in the forebrain, diagnosed in 1783

**Parkinson, James** (1755–1824); physician, England
  Parkinson's disease

**Rathke, Martin Heinrich** (1793–1860); anatomist, Germany
  Rathke's pouch

**Rolando, Luigi** (1773–1831); professor of anatomy, Turin
  Central (Rolandic) sulcus or fissure of Rolando: diagnosed in 1809

**Sylvius, Franciscus** (1614–1672); professor of practical medicine, Leyden, Amsterdam
  Aqueduct of Sylvius: connects the third and fourth ventricles, diagnosed in 1660
  Lateral Sylvian cerebral fissure: diagnosed in 1660

**Trolard, Paulin** (1842–1910); physician, Paris
  Vein of Trolard: diagnosed in 1868

**Wallenberg, Adolf** (1862–1949); neurologist, Germany
  Wallenberg's lateral medullary syndrome

**Wernicke, Karl** (1848–1905); neurologist, Germany
  Wernicke's area, fissure, triangle, dementia, encephalopathy, and aphasia

**Westphal Karl Friedrich Otto** (1833–1890); neurologist and psychiatrist, Berlin
  Edinger-Westphal nucleus

**Willis, Thomas** (1621–1675); physician, anatomist, and leader, London
  Circle of Willis: diagnosed in 1664

**Wilson, Samual Alaxander Kinnier** (1878–1937); neurologist, London
  Wilson's disease

# Index

Note: Page numbers in *italics* refer to illustrations.